D0908644

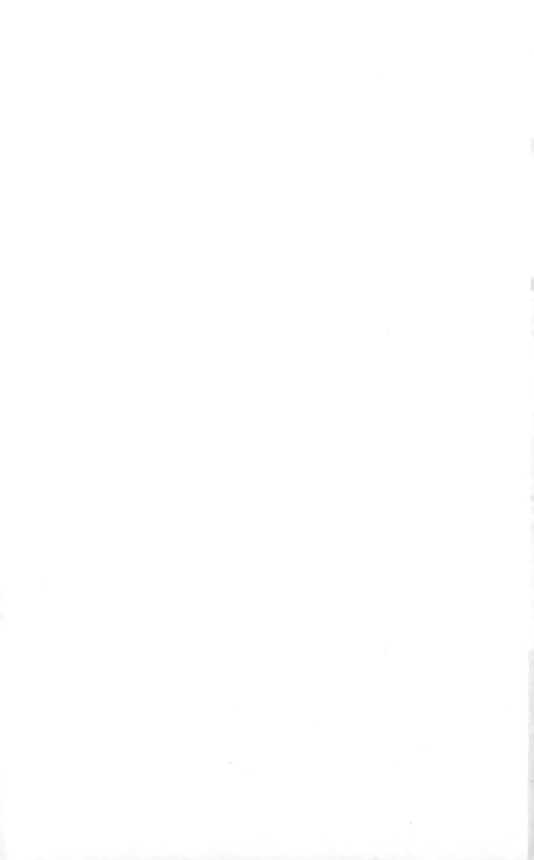

Family Partnership in Hospital Care

Anthony J. Grieco, MD, is Professor of Clinical Medicine at New York University School of Medicine, and Attending Physician in Medicine at Bellevue Hospital and Tisch Hospital. He is also Medical Director of the New York University Medical Center Cooperative Care Unit, a position he has held since 1979.

An alumnus of NYU and its School of Medicine, Dr. Grieco is co-editor, with Lawrence Bernstein and Mary Dete, of *Primary Care in the Home* and a member of the editorial board of *Staying Healthy in a Risky Environment*. He is medical editor of the WCBS Radio "Report on Medicine," which is heard throughout the New York metropolitan area, and of the Associated Press "Healthwire" series, which appears in newspapers and on radio stations across the country. In addition, he serves as a member of the Editorial Board of *Patient Education and Counseling* and as Medical Advisor to R *for Health*, which is published by NYU Medical Center.

Dr. Grieco is a Diplomate of the American Board of Internal Medicine, a Fellow of the American College of Physicians, and a member of the Society of General Internal Medicine. He also is a member of Phi Beta Kappa and Alpha Omega Alpha.

Margaret L. McClure, RN, EdD, is Vice President for Hospital Operations and Executive Director of Nursing at the New York University Medical Center in New York City, Adjunct Professor in the NYU Division of Nursing, where she teaches a graduate course in nursing administration, and Professor of Nursing Administration in the School of Medicine. She has been a member of the senior administration at NYU Medical Center since 1979 and has been involved in both the clinical and administrative aspects of NYU's Cooperative Care program since its inception.

Dr. McClure holds a Master of Arts in Nursing Service Administration and a Doctorate of Education from Teachers College of Columbia University.

A Fellow of the American Academy of Nursing and member and past President of the American Organization of Nurse Executives, she is internationally recognized as an authority in her field, serves on numerous advisory committees, and is the author of numerous publications.

Bruce K. Komiske, MHA, FACHE, is Executive Director of Hasbro Children's Hospital and the Rhode Island Hospital/Women and Infants Hospital Cooperative Care Center. Prior to his current position he served as Vice President of Planning, Marketing and Business Development at Rhode Island Hospital and President of RIH Ventures, a wholly owned subsidiary of the hospital created to develop and operate innovative health care businesses. In that capacity he developed the Cooperative Care Center and the Medical Mall in which it is located, and the Hasbro Children's Hospital. He orchestrated the development of "Steere House," a 120–bed geriatric center with no hospital equity, and was one of the founders of Health Advantage, a preferred provider organization comprised of 6 hospitals in Rhode Island which provides direct contracting for employee health care between the hospitals/physicians and the business community.

Prior to his arrival at Rhode Island Hospital in 1986, he served as Administrator of Norwood Hospital in Norwood, MA, and Vice President of Yale-New Haven Hospital in New Haven, CT.

An alumnus of the University of Pittsburgh, Mr. Komiske received a Master's Degree in Hospital Administration from Duke University. He is a Fellow of the American College of Health Care Executives and currently serves as a Regent for Rhode Island.

Robert F. Menard, FHFMA, is Senior Vice President for Corporate Development at Women and Infants Hospital in Providence, Rhode Island, a position he has held since 1986, and President of Palomar Group, Inc., a nonprofit venture company. Prior to his current position he was Associate Administrator at South County Hospital in South County, Rhode Island and held various positions at Coopers & Lybrand. He is an alumnus of Boston College, and a Fellow of the Healthcare Financial Management Association. Mr. Menard has served as an advisor to the Director of the Rhode Island State Department of Health. He is an active member of the Hospital Association of Rhode Island. Mr. Menard has been responsible for much of the financial planning for the Cooperative Care Center of Rhode Island and has been the senior representative from Women and Infants Hospital on the joint venture planning team.

Family Partnership in Hospital Care

The Cooperative Care Concept

Anthony J. Grieco, MD

Margaret L. McClure, RN, EdD, FAAN

Bruce K. Komiske, MHA, FACHE

Robert F. Menard, FHFMA

Editors

A New England Healthcare Assembly Book

 Springer Publishing Company

Copyright © 1994 by Springer Publishing Company, Inc.

Springer Publishing Company, Inc.
536 Broadway
New York, NY 10012

94 95 96 97 98 / 5 4 3 2 1

Library of Congress Cataloging-in-Publication Data

Family partnership in hospital care : the cooperative care concept /
  Anthony J. Grieco . . . [et al.] editors.
    p. cm.
  Includes bibliographical references and index.
  ISBN 0–8261–8490–1
  1. Cooperative care (Hospital care) 2. Cooperative care (Hospital
care)—United States. I. Grieco, Anthony J.
  [DNLM: 1. Patient Care Planning. 2. Hospital Administration.
3. Organizational Innovation. 4. Family. WX 162.5 1994]
RA965.6.F35 1994
362.1'1—dc20
DNLM/DLC
for Library of Congress   94-10518
                                                               CIP

Printed in the United States of America

CONTENTS

CONTRIBUTORS

Theresa A. Bischoff, MBA, CPA
Executive Vice President
NYU Medical Center
New York, NY

Pamela Brown, RN, MA
Director of Nursing for Risk
  Management and Quality
  Assurance
NYU Medical Center
New York, NY

Richard A. Browning, MD
Clinical Assistant Professor of
  Anesthesiology
Brown University School of
  Medicine,
Anesthesiologist-in-Chief
Rhode Island Hospital
Providence, RI

Rosalyn Cama, ASID
Rosalyn Cama Interior Design
  Associates, Inc.
New Haven, CT

James R. Carlson, AIA
Executive Vice President
The Robinson Green Geretta
  Corporation
Providence, RI

Esther Chachkes, MSW
Director of Social Services
NYU Medical Center
New York, NY

A. Judith Chwalow, RN, DrPH
Unite de Reserches Statisques
Villejuif, FRANCE

Rosemary Dale, RN, EdD
Vice President, Nursing and Patient
  Services
Medical Center Hospital of Vermont
Burlington, VT

Jeanne Dzurenko, RN, MPH
Head Nurse, Cooperative Care
NYU Medical Center
New York, NY

David S. Frieder, AIA
The Robinson Green Beretta
  Corporation
Providence, RI

Shirley Garnett, RN, MS
Former Manager of Education
  Center
Cooperative Care
NYU Medical Center
New York, NY

Kimberly S. Glassman, RN, MA
Director of Nursing Cooperative
  Care
NYU Medical Center
New York, NY

**Jeffrey B. Greene, MD, FACP,
  FCCP**
Clinical Associate Professor of
  Medicine
NYU Medical Center
New York, NY

Doreen M. Hackley, MS
Director, Department of Education
  and Training
Department of Human Resources
Rhode Island Hospital
Providence, RI

Diane Hanley, IBD
The Robinson Green Beretta
  Corporation
Providence, RI

Daniel D. Hanlon, BS
Human Resource Development
  Specialist
Rhode Island Hospital
Providence, RI

Richard H. Kennedy, MA, MBA
Vice President for Operations
Women & Infants Hospital
Providence, RI

May Kernan, BA
Vice Presidente/Group Manager
Potter-Hazelhurst Inc.
East Greenwich, RI

Theodore W. Kinkel, MBA, RD
Vice President, Regional Operations
Marriott Health Care Services
Franklin, MA

Bruce K. Komiske, MHA, FACHE
Executive Director
Hasbro Children's Hospital and
the Cooperative Care Center of
  Rhode Island
Providence, RI

Wanda Kowalski, RN, MA
Clinical Assistant Director of
  Nursing
NYU Medical Center
New York, NY

Richard Kuehl, AIA
The Robinson Green Beretta
  Corporation
Providence, RI

David M. Levine, MD, MPH, ScD
Director, Division of Internal
  Medicine
The Johns Hopkins University
School of Medicine
Baltimore, MD

Joyce Mamon, PhD
Treviso, ITALY

Margaret McClure, RN, EdD, FAAN
Vice President for Hospital Operations
and Executive Director of Nursing
NYU Medical Center
New York, NY

Sydney J. Mehl, MD, FACC
Clinical Associate Professor of Medicine
NYU Medical Center
New York, NY

Robert F. Menard, FHFMA
Senior Vice President for Corporate Development
Women & Infants Hospital
Providence, RI

Patricia Minuchin, PhD
Research Professor of Psychiatry
NYU Medical Center
New York, NY

Salvador Minuchin, MD
Research Professor of Psychiatry
NYU Medical Center
New York, NY

Christopher J. Morin, MD, MBA
Clinical Assistant Professor of Surgery
Brown University School of Medicine
Providence, RI

Grace Phelan, RN, MSN, MPA
Supervisor, Educator Center
Cooperative Care
NYU Medical Center
New York, NY

Jean Richards
New York, NY

Donald E. Schildkamp, MSIE
Senior Management Engineer
Rhode Island Hospital
Providence, RI

Florence S. Schumacher, MBA
Director of Marketing
Rhode Island Hospital
Providence, RI

Alan R. Schukman, RN, BSN
Clinical Coordinator, Cooperative Care
NYU Medical Center
New York, NY

Steven M. Sepe, MD, PhD
Associate Clinical Professor of Medicine
Brown University School of Medicine
Medical Director
Cooperative Care Center of Rhode Island
Providence, RI

James L. Speyer, MD
Associate Professor of Clinical Medicine
NYU Medical Center
New York, NY

Chrysanthe C. Stamoulis, RN, MBA, CNAA
Vice President Patient Services
and Chief Nursing Officer
Rhode Island Hospital
Providence, RI

Patricia L. Valoon, RN, MS
Senior Administrator
and Director of Nursing
NYU Medical Center
New York, NY

Kenneth Weiner, BM, BME
Senior Management Engineer
Rhode Island Hospital
Providence, RI

Irvin G. Wilmot, MBA, LFACHE
Professor of Health Care
   Management
Former Executive Vice President
NYU Medical Center
New York, NY

PREFACE

Imagine a hospital where patients stay in private rooms with a family member, rooms to which they have the key; where patients wear their own clothes rather than hospital "johnnies"; where patients visit the physicians and nurses, rather than vice versa. Imagine a hospital where family "care partners" help in the physical care of the patient, giving medications, and observing changes in condition that might be missed by a busy nurse; where family members and patients attend health education classes together and eat together in a cafeteria.

This form of hospital care is called "cooperative care" and it has been successfully implemented in a 104-patient unit at New York University Medical Center since 1979. Cooperative care is the direct involvement of the family, be it traditional or nontraditional, in the hospital care of a family member. Patients selected for the unit must have a willing and available "care partner," as the family member is called. A wide range of patients have been successfully treated in this unit, including people with AIDS, cardiovascular disease, and cancer. As a result of the cooperative care program, patients are less isolated and less afraid during their hospital stay and they have more of a sense of control over their environment. Further, family members are better prepared to take over necessary caring functions when the patient returns home. The care is of high quality, and results in fewer mishaps, such as mistakes in medication and falling out of bed. Cooperative care is cost effective as well; it is nearly a third less costly than traditional hospital care.

This book describes cooperative care from both conceptual and applied perspectives. Part I, the bulk of the book, provides an in-depth look at the concepts and programs developed at NYU Medical Center. Part II gives an insiders view of the planning for the second major implementation of cooperative care, at the Cooperative Care Center of Rhode Island, which is scheduled to open in July, 1994.

This book was written to share the experience of NYU Medical Center and Rhode Island Hospital/Women and Infants Hospital with interested health care professionals and administrators. We hope that more institutions and caregivers will be stimulated to create their own versions of this humane and effective method of hospital care.

A CARE PARTNER'S PERSPECTIVE

NYU Medical Center
530 First Avenue
New York, NY 10016

Dear Sir or Madam:

My mother and I spent a week or so in Cooperative Care recently, and on her behalf, I want to thank you. It was a wonderful experience, for both her (the patient) and me. I had peace of mind because I was with her, not subject to the bureaucratic and rigid visitation hours, wondering if she was getting the right medicine, unnecessary tests, or not enough observation.

Not having to sit at home, wondering how she was feeling, but being able to be there with her and help her myself.

The simplest way I can describe her pleasure in Cooperative Care, besides the company of a caring daughter, was that she was treated as an adult. This sounds obvious, but it's not. Only when one contrasts Cooperative Care with regular hospital care does one realize that in a hospital one is treated as a child, and not even a very intelligent child, at that.

It is deeply satisfying, and very unusual to be accorded the respect one deserves as an intelligent adult, in a hospital setting. This respect ranges from trusting that you can take the right medicine at the right time, to addressing you by your last name (No "Hi Eva, I'm Jane"), to allowing both caregiver and patient to use their own good judgment regarding daily life questions (no "lights out at 9 P.M.," "no visitors under 12," etc.). Only a stay at Cooperative Care highlights the condescension with which one is treated in regular care, for the sake of hospital efficiency.

Thank you for this wonderful, innovative (though ancient in other cultures) concept. I hope for the sake of other families that it will take root in many hospitals across the country.

Sincerely,
Jean Richards
New York, NY

ACKNOWLEDGMENTS

Sincere thanks to the staff of NYU Medical Center's Cooperative Care unit over the past 15 years, who are the indirect contributors to this book. Special thanks, particularly to two people: Elizabeth Kramer, without whose stimulus, as well her conceptual and editorial skills, this book might not have existed; and Delores Debnam, whose patience, persistence, and endurance enabled our ideas to become a completed manuscript.

PART I
The Who, What, Why, and How of Cooperative Care

1

ORIGINS OF COOPERATIVE CARE

Anthony J. Grieco, Kimberly S. Glassman, and
Shirley A. Garnett

PROBLEMS WITH TRADITIONAL HOSPITAL CARE

Hospitalization is a hazardous proposition for many people, particularly for the elderly (Creditor, 1993), who often leave the hospital with less independence, less mobility, and less capability than was their situation prior to admission. Although this is commonly the result of the natural history of the disease which prompted the hospital stay, or due to the expected need for recuperation after major surgery, in many instances the deterioration in level of function at home following hospitalization is not explainable by these factors.

What are the dangers which hospitalization itself holds for the elderly, compounding the risks they face from their illnesses? First of all, hospitals put people in bed, keeping them at rest almost routinely, thereby deconditioning muscle strength, and respiratory capacity, provoking postural hypotension, and advancing osteoporosis. If the patient is bedridden and without adequate minute-to-minute personal attention, urinary incontinence may be unavoidable. This can accelerate skin breakdown, leading to decubitus ulceration. Lacking around-the-clock presence of close family members eliminates those who are the most helpful in preventing confusion and agitation. Nutrition may suffer if feeding requires time-consuming patience which may demand more time than is available to nurses and nurse-aides. According to a study by Creditor (1993) of problems of a geriatric population during hospitalization, and of their solutions, the negative impact of hospitalization upon the level of function begins immediately upon admission and continues to progress at a relatively rapid pace throughout the stay.

Is this decline in functional ability unavoidable? Are there any strategies for blunting hospitalization's negative impact? A start can be made by making the hospital more homelike in ways which do not adversely affect the safety inherently needed during the time of acute illness. For example, Creditor (1993) recommends that bed rest be avoided whenever it is not truly essential. Hospital beds can be kept at their lowest height, eliminating the need for bedrails. Traction can be improved by using carpeting, thereby reducing falls. Intravenous lines can be kept capped except when a therapeutic infusion is being administered. Lighting can be bright during daytime and very soft at night.

Hospitals also can learn from the experiences of nursing homes, which encourage patients to wear their own personal clothing and to share mealtimes as social occasions, rather than as solitary bedside events. A partnership also should be created among the interdisciplinary care-providing professionals. Creditor (1993) asserts that the therapeutic value to be gained from these seemingly minor steps can be as important as the benefits of the prescribed treatment regimen itself.

PATIENT-ORIENTED VS. HEALTHCARE WORKER-ORIENTED CARE

The notions just described are consistent with the concept of "the kindly stress of hospitalization," a term coined by Bedell, Cleary, and DelBanco (1984). They identified generally accepted hospital policies and procedures which are detrimental to patients' response to illness, and which actually impede recovery. They found that rather than encouraging the change in lifestyle that would help to modify the long-term outcome of the disease process, the experience of being hospitalized may, in some instances, actually interfere with the individual's ability to adapt appropriately to the needed changes. In part, this is due to the dependency forced upon people by restrictive hospital regulations which control so many aspects of a patient's daily life. During the usual hospital confinement, responsibility for selection of diet, personal attire, and scheduling of the day's events are entirely the prerogative of the hospital staff. Patients give up these rights, as well as privacy, in the name of safety. Doors are kept open, semi-open hospital gowns are commonly used, and hospital personnel peer in uninvited and give instructions which are designated as "orders," not requests. As an outgrowth of this authoritarian scene, patients may feel coerced into accepting medical decisions passively, often while being under informed, rather than achieving a partnership role in the medical decision making process.

Bedell, Cleary, and DelBanco (1984) advocate developing an alternate model of care. Their model would give patients a fuller awareness of the activities and habits that enhance or retard healing and health. It would stimulate people to assume an active role in their own care. People would be encouraged to learn strategies that would enable them to better cope with the disease or condition after they leave the hospital. They propose changing the focus of care in hospitals, making it more patient-centered. They further propose that patients become active partners with professionals as participants in care, rather than merely being recipients of care. They promote involving patients fully in decisions, putting a major effort into educating patients completely about their illness, and teaching them the skills necessary to collect their own meaningful information independently. They feel that this would enable patients to anticipate the problems they might confront after discharge from the hospital, and to become capable of developing their own strategies for dealing with them. They argue that this active involvement by patients in their own care will result not only in more effective care, but in more humane care as well.

SHARING RESPONSIBILITY: PATIENT AND FAMILY PARTNERSHIP IN CARE

Perhaps this degree of involvement in care can result in what has been called "a new stage in health care—the era of the patient"(Reiser, 1993, p. 1012), leading to a true partnership in care. The partnership can extend beyond that of doctor and patient, or of health care professionals and patient. The family should be brought into this partnership as well, as noted by the Council on Scientific Affairs of the American Medical Association (Council on Scientific Affairs, 1993).

The Council (1993), acknowledging that family members play a most essential and central role in managing home care, notes that family members themselves provide at least 80% of the home health care received by frail elderly people. Approximately two-thirds of the responsible family members are women (a spouse or daughter), as noted in other studies. What duties do these family members perform? Providing assistance with activities of daily living was at the top of the list, including help with grooming, feeding, dressing, toileting, transferring, and ambulating.

Long-term responsibility for providing care to a disabled family member at home did have some measurable negative impact upon the physical and emotional wellbeing of those providing the care. This was true even in those circumstances in which the family member willingly undertook the care, and even when providing care gave the individual personal pleasure. The factors which had the greatest negative impact upon the caring family were incontinence of urine or stool, particularly when the patient had dementia. In those circumstances, the family members were more likely to become less tolerant, lose their sense of commitment, and to perceive their own health, confidence and competence as deteriorating.

How can these negatives be avoided or overcome? The Council recommends (1993) that the degree of functioning of the patient-family team be kept under observation and in focus by the professionals, who should note their interactions and interdependencies, and who should make decisions for care in this context. This kind of focus and attention is thought to result in better outcomes for both the patient and the family member responsible for care. The Council recommends providing specific education and training for family caregivers so that they can be better equipped to handle their challenges. It also recommends that the responsible family caregiver be encouraged to seek help from other family members for relief whenever possible.

A family care partner's view of participating in a patient's illness has been most eloquently expressed recently by a man writing of "our breast cancer," describing how he and his wife dealt with that diagnosis and its treatment options (Dodge, 1993, p. 20). His participation in care appeared to be of enormous help to both of them:

> She wasn't really sure that everything would be all right between us until we got home and she had to submit to my fumbling with the bandages on the wound and on the drain. There's a lot of talk about moral support groups but she told me that just the fiddling with the dressings was a greater and more loving proof of support than any of those people could possibly offer or dream of. (p. 20)

COST CONSIDERATIONS IN HOSPITALIZATION

"The inflationary spiral of health care costs" is not a new phenomenon; it was considered the virtual by-word of the seventies. However, since that time there has been little change in the manner of health delivery which holds promise of breaking this pattern.

Most cost-containment efforts have been focused on doing with less: less staff, fewer specialists, reduced supplies, lower ancillaries, and reduced bed complement. All of these are geared toward eliminating an assumed element of waste from the providers of health care. As initial steps they were important; there is no questioning the need to reduce excesses in the system. These efforts, however, fall short of any long-term solution because once the system is "de-fatted," business is essentially being done in the same way.

The approaches which must be encouraged and expanded are those aimed at substantive change in health care delivery. Appropriately, those efforts have been targeted at the acute hospital facility, since expenditures for hospitals are the largest component of the health care dollar (Sommers, 1971). Most efforts have been epitomized by developments, like ambulatory surgery centers, which serve as alternatives to expensive inpatient care.

New York University Medical Center has pioneered a new concept in health care delivery which brings the alternate delivery efforts to full maturity. Its Cooperative Care Center, which opened in April 1979, marked a true health care breakthrough which couples improved patient care with creative cost containment. Rather than seeking an alternative to acute care, it changed the very nature of the hospital itself.

THE COOPERATIVE CARE CONCEPT

For acute patients admitted to Cooperative Care, the days spent in the unit substitute for those that previously would have been spent in traditional hospital beds. The Cooperative Care program requires that patients be joined by a care partner—a family member, friend or companion—who assumes responsibility for the patient's personal care and routine bedside needs, in the way those needs would be met at home. Both the patient and care partner participate in an intensive disease-specific educational program structured to help them cope with the patient's illness and modified state of health. This care team of patient and care partner has an opportunity to function under the supervision of professional personnel, and begin a meaningful transition to home prior to actual discharge.

The Cost Impacts Of Cooperative Care

In essence, the Cooperative Care concept is two fold. The program strives to tailor the care environment to the current needs of the patient, and to improve the patient's ability to deal with the realities of postdischarge existence. These concepts join to attack the causes of high cost health care on several fronts.

The Cooperative Care program has an impact on the cost of health care by:

- reducing the cost of hospitalization;
- maximizing the use of limited resources; and
- reducing the incidence of additional episodes of institutional care.

The most immediate of these impacts are felt solely within the parent institution, New York University Medical Center. The secondary ones have significant consequences for the entire health care delivery system.

Reduction in the Cost of Hospitalization

Probably the most immediate impact of Cooperative Care is a reduction in the cost of hospitalization. The Center's opening meant that a portion of certain patients' care can be provided in a less costly environment, reducing the average cost of a hospital stay.

Specifically, Cooperative Care is able to provide patient services at approximately two-thirds of the cost of New York University's traditional acute facility. This cost reduction is achieved because all aspects of Cooperative Care are designed to limit the potential impact of two of the major factors of hospital costs: hospital staffing, and construction and equipment requirements.

Labor: Its Unique Role in Health Care

By its nature, health care is a labor-intensive industry; more than two-thirds of most hospital budgets are expended on personnel (Metzger & Panter, 1972). This has been true from the time when medical practice was little more than hand holding. What often goes unrecognized, however, is that increased technology has actually served to intensify the human factor in health care costs.

Many major developments in our ability to manage disease are accomplished by the generation of new breeds of technicians. In fact, the medical science knowledge explosion of the last decades has resulted in an increased staffing complement per acute hospital bed of 171% (Metzger & Panter, 1972). The corresponding impact on hospital costs has been staggering.

Increased specialization of labor, and ever-rising numbers of professional and support staffs, mean that any development in health care delivery which limits traditional areas of labor dependency will realize reduced costs. Cooperative Care does exactly this.

Staffing Needs in Cooperative Care

Traditionally, high-risk diagnostic procedures and the initial stages of recuperation have had to take place in an acute hospital. This was often not because of the care the patient *did* need, but rather because of the care the patient *might* need. With its direct physical link to the services of the traditional acute hospital units, Cooperative Care provides only those services consistent with the actual needs of patients. The ramifications for staffing are dramatic.

Appropriate candidate selection is pivotal to the success of the Cooperative Care program. Among other criteria, mobility status (including those patients who use locomotion aids, such as canes, crutches, walkers or wheelchairs) is a prerequisite for admission to Cooperative Care. Once admitted to the unit, patients go to a centralized therapeutic center for assessment and treatments, and take their meals in a central dining room. They have scheduled physician and treatment appointments, as well as comprehensive educational sessions.

The "carer" aspect of the partner's role further augments traditional staffing patterns for recuperating patients. In this system, professional nursing care is administered predominantly in the centralized therapeutic center.

These arrangements dramatically reduce the need for patients to be in full-time direct view of the professional staff. Cooperative Care's reduced staffing realizes immediate cost savings. Perhaps even more important, though, is that the fundamental concept of Cooperative Care minimizes traditional dependence on an expensive and volatile factor in the health care cost equation.

Construction: The Forgotten Cost

The same forces of modern technology which have changed the composition of health care labor have made themselves felt in the hospital's physical environment. The physical specifications of a baseline acute unit are filled with medical advances which necessitate high costs. Diagnostic developments have dictated the installation of transport systems to assure the speedy delivery of specimens to the laboratory. For example, minutes count in the processing of blood gases on immediately postoperative cardiac patients. Strides in infection control have generated complex ventilation systems, now standard for acute hospitals.

As is the case with its staffing pattern, the physical environment of the acute hospital is adjusted to handle the most difficult phase of the care of the traditional acute hospital patient. The costs of these selectively used features affect all phases of the stay.

By structuring the environment for the current needs of its unique patient population, Cooperative Care realizes sizeable cost savings. Bereft of bedside oxygen and the like, the hotel-type Cooperative Care rooms have been built for a fraction of the cost of standard hospital construction. In addition, the need for future modernization is minimal, as Cooperative Care programs are largely impervious to most innovations in medical technology. Of course, innovations in health education are constantly incorporated into Cooperative Care's program, but there has been no need for significant structural change.

Allocation of Resources

The introduction of a Cooperative Care-like facility into a medical center complex has widespread repercussions in the existing acute units. Potentially, the most significant of these is the effect on the patient mix, especially with regard to acuity level and intensity of service.

With the addition of 104 Cooperative Care beds, the Medical Center assures that only those patients requiring and utilizing the specialized services of an acute hospital are occupying it. From a generic cost containment perspective, therefore, Cooperative Care results in a more efficient allocation of the expensive services basic to a standard acute hospital. This allocation is necessary to achieve the most efficient use of the health care system's finite resources.

Reduction in Additional Episodes of Institutional Care

The cost-saving features of Cooperative Care include significant system-wide economies, achieved by segregating appropriate patients into a unit devoid of those now-superfluous services, and maximizing their use in the standard acute area. This, however, is only part of Cooperative Care's cost containment effect.

On this cost-saving foundation of eliminated services, the Cooperative Care program builds additional long-term economies by addressing the unique clinical needs of its selected acute care patients. These needs extend far beyond the physical process of healing. Patients with an acute illness episode have a very real need to mend mentally and emotionally. Although lip service is given to social and emotional needs of patients, the hospital continues to reflect the priority given to the technical-scientific aspects of the medical role (Mechanic, 1968). Even with the "miracles of modern medicine," a total return to pre-hospital health status is often impossible. In these instances, it is particularly crucial that the new health equilibrium include both a physical and a psychological component.

Not only are these needs rarely fully met in a traditional acute care hospital, but the structure and concepts of the institution are essentially at odds with them. Sociologists have found that there are many analogies which can be drawn between the hospital and other bureaucratic organizations; among them, there is a tendency to try to limit client control (Mechanic, 1968). The responsibility for this lies not with the acute hospital but, rather, with its present multifaceted role in the health care delivery system.

Despite all that is known about the complexities of acute care, the unrealistic expectation that the hospital can effectively be all things to all types of acute patients remains. Of course, it cannot.

Rather, the limited resources of the acute hospital are appropriately keyed to those patients with the greatest needs; i.e., those in the most unstable phase of their illness. Researchers have found that patients actually limit the expression of their needs for personalized and supportive care because they perceive that it is superseded by other patients' need for physical care (Tagliacozzo & Mauksch, 1972). The best of intentions do not change the fact that little professional time is available for patient teaching.

The sociological environment also is structured for the most critical patients. When imposed on other patients, the supportive hospital atmosphere fosters unnecessary dependency.

The acute hospital often cannot effectively provide fundamental information concerning the patient's changed state of health or an opportunity for patient and family to deal with it. This failure is visited upon the health care system in the form of increased posthospital extended care placements and a high incidence of rehospitalization.

The Cooperative Care Program

The Cooperative Care program realizes its full cost containment potential by effecting long-term economies through reducing the causes of expensive inpatient care. The needs of the patient are met through both a formal education program and a targeted environment.

The noninstitutional environment of Cooperative Care provides a *de facto* mechanism for addressing the patient's need for secure independence. The hotel-type rooms are free of hospital gadgetry which tend to reinforce feelings of dependency and illness. Allowing the patients to wear street clothing, the absence of artificially imposed schedules for care regimens, and the normalized dining facilities create an environment in which patients can be treated without suffering the womblike hospital atmosphere of usual hospital units.

The care partner, too, can make the difficult transition from hospital to home with the availability of professional staff support. The opportunity to perform care regimens in semi-independence minimizes the anxiety usually associated with taking a partially dependent patient home.

Coupled with this controlled opportunity to deal with the patient's modified state of health, Cooperative Care's program provides the patient and care partner with the necessary information to do so on an intelligent basis.

Cost-Effective Patient Education

During their stay at Cooperative Care, both members of the care team participate in an intensive, disease-specific education program.

Cooperative Care's capacity to individualize the education program is illustrative of New York University Medical Center's efforts to capitalize on principles which have proven effective in other health education efforts. It should be noted that despite the expanding national commitment to the concepts of health education (Sommers, 1978), these remain major issues of debate. Although the connection between behavior and health outcomes has been firmly established (Sommers, 1978), controversy centers on the most effective way of modifying behavior.

Of all the types of health education (including school health education, occupational health education, national programs, community health education, and media programs) patient education has proven the most successful (Sommers & Sommers, 1977). Clearly, motivation to effect a change is at a high point when a person is experiencing the undesirable patient role (Mechanic, 1968). Cooperative Care, therefore, effects a true health conversion, because it intervenes at a critical moment: during an acute illness episode.

Evidence also suggests that to impact lifestyles, a person must receive "highly targeted health messages" (Green, 1977, p. 160). By

tailoring the health education modules to the patient, Cooperative
Care's program has the advantage of addressing very specific behavior
patterns.

A final aspect of Cooperative Care which promises success is its controlled, yet independent, environment. This atmosphere, on the one
hand, allows the patient to start to make certain choices which can
impact health status and, on the other hand, provides positive reinforcement for appropriate choices. This social reinforcement has been
recognized as vital in effecting long-term life style change (Sommers,
1978).

The success of a health education program can be evaluated in
terms of actual reductions in health care expenditures. From a global
perspective, studies have shown that changes in behavior are associated with a reduction in the incidence of certain diseases (Sommers &
Sommers, 1977). Such disease avoidance means the elimination of
costs entailed in their treatment, as well as the elimination of cost to
the national economy involved in work absenteeism and disability
(Klarman, 1974).

Perhaps even more important, evidence now indicates the potential
for short-term savings from patient education. These savings are
emerging in the form of changed inpatient utilization patterns. In
terms of Cooperative Care, they are achieved from fewer extended care
placements, due to the increased competence and confidence of the patient and family, and a general reduction in rehospitalization. Improved self-care patterns and diminished anxiety after patient education are in part responsible for this reduction in rehospitalization. The
results in this area have been very hopeful: one study found a reduction in rehospitalization of 90% (Sommers & Sommers, 1977). Of
course, expectations of this magnitude are unrealistic. The hard evidence does indicate, however, that Cooperative Care realizes significant savings through reduced extended care and rehospitalization.

THE AMERICAN HOSPITAL IN TOMORROW'S
HEALTH CARE DELIVERY

If the hospital is to survive in a meaningful fashion, it must adapt to
the evolving environment of American health care. Increasingly, this
environment is marked by limited resources and a changed philosophy. The dominant position has shifted from efforts focused purely on
medical care to those concerned with health care, with an enlarged
role for personal responsibility.

In this adaptation process, the Cooperative Care Center serves as a vital link between what the American hospital has been and what it can become. To accomplish the necessary transition, the traditional paradigms which have governed health care delivery must be abandoned. Encased in standard logic, the hospital is doomed to ever-expanding costs and a shrinking ability to meet the broad health care needs of the American people.

Cooperative Care explodes the parochialism that has hampered development of delivery alternatives. In so doing, it reaps savings from simplified staffing and construction, reduced placement and rehospitalization, and maximization of acute services.

These savings, the essence of the Cooperative Care concept, are representative of the kind of creative cost containment needed to equip the American health delivery system for the challenges of the 21st century.

2

HOW DOES COOPERATIVE CARE WORK? AN OVERVIEW

Anthony J. Grieco, Kimberly S. Glassman,
Shirley A. Garnett, and Grace Phelan

BACKGROUND PLANNING

The Cooperative Care Unit of New York University (NYU) Medical
Center opened in April, 1979, the first of its kind in the world. The
unit was 15 years in its planning (Astolfi & Wilmot, 1972), with involvement by representatives of the federal, state, and local health authorities and the local Blue Cross plan, in conjunction with the Medical Center's trustees, administration, faculty, and staff. Cooperative
Care grew out of a quest for a way to utilize the advantages gained
from patient education to provide a higher level of care to acute care
hospital inpatients, without consuming the same volume of expensive

professional and technical resources required by traditional hospital units.

The idea began by evaluating the desirability of organizing the hospital along the lines of stratified levels of care, ranging from intensive care units to step-down units and self-care units. However, lower level care units subsequently were eliminated from consideration as unworkable, since such units would not provide sufficient care for seriously ill inpatients.

How, then, would it become possible to provide enhanced patient care with lower hospital resource consumption? Identifying the cost of personnel and staffing—the primary rate-limiting factor in the provision of a high level of care—and facing the reality that acutely ill inpatients cannot be relied upon to safely provide their own self-care, the family members and friends who provided home care prior to hospitalization and following discharge were studied for their potential availability as participants in care during the hospital stay itself.

With hospitalization looked upon as a relatively brief interlude in a life spent predominantly at home, it became apparent that the family members or friends who are responsible for any needed physical assistance and emotional support, observation, assistance with treatments, administration of medications, and help with feeding, as well as being available to call for additional professional help when required at home (Bernstein, Dete, & Grieco, 1985; Grieco & Kowalski, 1987; Wadsworth & Grieco, 1987) would likely be capable of performing similar functions in an inpatient setting, if they were reasonably comfortably accommodated.

Of course, home life and hospital care are quite different from one another. Hospital care has a much finer focus on acute illness, while home care has a broader, longer-term agenda. Hospital care generates a great deal of directly measured technical data, while home care has little technical data but much more family-observed personal data. Hospital care has extensive, and expensive, resources, while home care has limited resources available. Hospital care has a professional caring team, while home care has only the family and patient, and occasionally a temporarily hired aide or companion. With its high-tech and extensive resources, however, the hospital provides more "generic" care, in that the staff work for the hospital, not for the individual patient, and any specific patient's needs must be weighed in priority against competing demands upon the staff's time. Home care, by contrast, provides patient-specific care. Thus, incorporating a family member as part of the hospital team would actually raise the level of patient-specific care, broaden its agenda, and provide family-observed personal data which would otherwise be unavailable in the inpatient setting.

This is the groundwork upon which Cooperative Care was created. It became an acute hospital unit of 104 patient rooms with a homelike setting, incorporating for each patient a living-in family member or friend, called a "care partner," who shares responsibility with the hospital staff, actively participating in care, observation, and treatment. Oral medications generally are administered by the care partner. This is preceded by detailed instruction given by a pharmacist and nurse-educator, with validation of the reliability of this care by the clinical nurse who oversees the management while handling the more technical diagnostic and therapeutic interventions. The living area of the unit is separated from the area of core services in which the nurses and other hospital staff are located. This physical separation heightens the patient's and family's awareness of the necessity to quickly develop a deeper understanding of the disease, as well as proficiency in semi-autonomous care.

It quickly became obvious that utilizing a family member or friend as a care partner during hospitalization truly provided one-on-one observation of the patient, even when the professional staff were not on the scene, and the active family presence dramatically lowered the number of professional staff members required, thus substantially dropping the cost of hospitalization without reducing quality of care. The cost savings was predicted to be (Astolfi & Wilmot, 1972), and actually has continued to be, one-third of the cost of the usual hospital care.

OBJECTIVES OF COOPERATIVE CARE

Three objectives were identified in designing the Cooperative Care program:

1. reduction of the cost of acute care hospitalization by caring for patients in the unit most suited to their needs, utilizing as manpower the combined efforts of the patient and family member or friend;

2. decrease in the likelihood of rehospitalization by having the patient and care partner effectively learn to deal with the illness through active participation in care, supplemented by a comprehensive health education program; and

3. increase in the availability of the resources of the traditional part of the hospital for more intensive care needs.

DESCRIPTION OF COOPERATIVE CARE

Cooperative Care is an integral part of the 726–bed Tisch Hospital of NYU Medical Center. The unit contains 104 patient rooms, each containing two beds: one for the patient, and the other for the care partner, who remains in the hospital accompanying and assisting the patient throughout the stay. The care partner's presence is the hallmark of the unit, and makes Cooperative Care capable of handling a diverse population of acutely ill medical patients (Grieco, 1987). Care partner and patient are lodged together in a homelike, two-bed, one-patient room on one of the five patient-room floors ("Cooperative care," 1981; Planck, 1982). The nurses, nurse-aides, physicians, and other staff are not assigned to roam those floors as they would be in a traditional hospital unit. Instead, the professional staff are concentrated in the centralized core services area above the patient-room floors. Rather than having hospital services delivered to their bedside, Cooperative Care patients come to the centralized clinical, educational, and dining services with the assistance of the care partner. Thus, most of the clinical nursing assessments and care, physician examinations and treatments, individual and group educational sessions, and meals are provided not at the bedside, but in the core services area. This leaves the patient-room floors remarkably free of the controlling influence which the hospital professionals exert ubiquitously in almost all inpatient settings.

Two of the traditional nursing functions, clinical care and patient education, are divided in Cooperative Care into two separate, but interdependent, sub-units: the "Therapeutic Center" for the clinical duties and the "Education Center" for teaching, each with its own defined staff. The combined efforts of the two sub-units empower the family members or friends who are acting in the role of care partners for their patients to assume a great deal of shared responsibility for personal care and observation, so that acutely ill patients with a wide variety of diseases can receive a higher level of care than is delivered in most traditional medical-surgical nursing units (Bernstein et al., 1985; Grieco, 1988; "Patient education," 1981).

The Education Center

The Education center is staffed by health professionals from four different disciplines: nurse education, nutrition, social work, and pharmacy (Kristan, 1985; Stark, 1987).

Nurse-educators begin the teaching process at the time of admission into Cooperative Care by obtaining the clinical history; assessing the clinical appropriateness of the patient; determining the adequacy of the care partner; orienting the patient and care partner to the Cooperative Care environment; and giving them detailed instructions regarding the responsibilities they will be called upon to perform during their stay. If the care partner appears inadequate to the tasks at hand, the nurse-educator, in conjunction with the social worker, is responsible for initiating basic instruction, giving emotional support and counseling, and for arranging to have the family or friend care partner supplemented, if needed, by a hired companion. An educational plan is generated, fitting together the perceived needs of the patient and care partner with the anticipated length of stay; setting priorities for relative importance of the various topics to be covered; and the urgency or timeliness of these topics with respect to the procedures and treatments planned by the physician.

The Education Center staff also are responsible for developing new educational programs, periodically updating existing lesson plans and handouts, and for linking patient educational strategies with other nursing units of NYU Medical Center. In addition, the Education Center provides a variety of outpatient health education programs, many of which are unrelated to the spectrum of teaching which is directed at Cooperative Care inpatients.

The patient and care partner education programs of Cooperative Care are designed to achieve the goals of increasing understanding of the disease process and its treatment regimen, and facilitating active participation by the patient/care partner team in the caring process during hospitalization.

Equally important, the education program stimulates continued compliance with the appropriate therapeutic and preventive measures advocated after discharge. This includes the expectation that health care resources, such as emergency room visits, will be used with good judgement following hospitalization; for example, that elective visits to the physician will be favored over emergent, episodic care.

An attempt is made by the educational staff to identify disease risk factors which can be controlled or modified. The nutritionists are particularly active in this area, since they need to meet and discuss food selection with the patient and care partner if a therapeutic diet is advised. This is more important to patients in this setting than to those in traditional medical-surgical hospital units, since in the Cooperative Care dining room patients select food cafeteria-style; they need to have the knowledge to choose the proper foods as they would at home or in a restaurant, rather than rely upon the hospital to provide a pre selected tray of food for them.

Overall, these educational measures have an effect not only of improving technical aspects of knowledge regarding treatment, but also have a measurable impact on improving patient satisfaction and in reducing anxiety of both the patient and family (Grieco, 1985).

The Therapeutic Center

Following the initial educational assessment at the Education Center, the patient and care partner undergo a clinical assessment by a nurse-clinician at the Therapeutic Center. This begins in much the traditional mode of examination, initial testing, medication administration, and scheduling of further diagnostic and therapeutic maneuvers. But, in addition to these functions, the nurse-clinician has the responsibility to prepare the patient and care partner for participation in care. For example, oral medications are likely to be dispensed to the patient/care partner team for administration by them in the patient room, after education has been provided and a solid level of understanding has been assured.

The Therapeutic Center is comprised of individual examining rooms, which look much like a physician's office or clinic. Patients and care partners are scheduled for follow up visits in these examining rooms at intervals determined by their clinical needs. Intravenous infusions, for example, might warrant visits with the nurse-clinician at 6-hour intervals.

A six-bed observation unit, which is part of the Therapeutic Center, is used as an area for more continuous nursing attention, in much the same manner as a recovery room or Intensive Care Unit. This site is used as a temporary location for patients who have just undergone potentially hazardous procedures, or who have been judged by the professional staff to appear clinically unstable. They stay there anywhere from one to several hours. Syncope, chest pain, arrhythmias, bleeding, seizures, or very high fever are some of the indications for temporarily placing patients into this location. After stabilization, the patient is "promoted" back to the Cooperative Care patient room with the care partner. Of course, in those instances in which the need for this level of care is protracted, the patient usually is transferred to the traditional Intensive Care Unit, as would be any patient from elsewhere in the medical center.

Opening Projections

In anticipation of the opening of Cooperative Care planned to occur in April, 1979, a study (Cooperative Care patient survey, unpublished data) was performed in 1976 and 1977 in the traditional medical-surgical units of NYU Medical Center. Its purpose was to evaluate the patient population with an eye toward identifying the potential volume and types of people who would be eligible for care when the new unit opened.

The three primary assumptions ("Draft Document," 1978) which were the underpinning for that study were that, first, Cooperative Care would provide an environment suitable for patients who require hospitalization without necessarily needing to utilize the entire spectrum of the services and facilities of the traditional units; second, that these patients would benefit from comprehensive health education directed at both the patient and family; and third, that the days the patient would be in Cooperative Care would otherwise have been days in the traditional hospital's nursing units.

The criteria used for identifying potential candidates for Cooperative Care were simply that the patient would require hospitalization; that the patient would be mobile, either independently or with assistance from the care partner; that direct nursing contact would likely not be needed more frequently than at 6-hour intervals; that the patient would be able to come to the Therapeutic Center for assessments and treatments; and that the patient's nursing needs could be handled by intermittent professional nurse attention, rather than requiring continuous bedside nursing care.

In performing the study, nurses gauged the patients in the hospital on survey days against the list of criteria just enumerated, selecting only those who met every criterion. They then retrospectively judged the day of the hospitalization on which the patient first met the criteria and could have been transferred to Cooperative Care, had it then been in existence, and calculated what the total length of stay in the unit would have been.

The study found that the patients who met criteria averaged 55 years in age. The length of stay in Cooperative Care was predicted to be half that of the total hospitalization, but since it was expected that the eligible patients would have high total hospital stay, the calculated Cooperative Care average length of stay was anticipated to be approximately 10 days.

In looking at the clinical services, the researchers predicted that the greatest number of patients would be on the medical service, which was predicted to account for 19% of the eligible patients. This was followed by the general surgical service and the urology service, each of which was expected to account for 15% of the eligible patients. The dermatology service would provide 11%, cardiology 9%, orthopedics and neurosurgery each 8%, and gynecology 5%, while the services of plastic surgery and otolaryngology each would account for 4% percent. Ophthalmology was predicted to account for just under 2% and psychiatry just over 1%, with neurology, pediatrics and radiology each predicted to provide less than 1% of eligible patients.

As far as the predicted diagnostic mix, malignancy was at the top, expected to account for 23% of the patients, followed by cardiovascular diseases as an additional 16%. Genitourinary disorders were predicted at 10%, dermatological disorders and digestive diseases each at 8% and musculoskeletal disorders at 6%. Neurological and endocrine disorders were predicted to account for only 4% each, and infectious diseases and respiratory disorders only about 2% each. Of course, these early predictions must be interpreted not only in the context of the hospitalization pattern of the seventies, but also with the realization that acquired immunodeficiency syndrome did not yet exist in the United States.

The study also made assumptions regarding whether the patient would be likely to enter Cooperative Care directly from home or be transferred from other medical-surgical nursing units of the medical center. Since the study utilized patients who were already hospitalized, it is not surprising that it predicted a larger number of transfers than direct admissions. However, predicted transfers only slightly edged the direct admissions, 53.5% to 46.5%. The study also predicted that a sizeable proportion of the Cooperative Care patients would be transferred to the traditional hospital nursing units rather than remaining in the new unit for the entire hospitalization. It was anticipated that nearly half of the direct admissions would move over to traditional care, but that only about 5% of the patients transferred from traditional care would be retransferred back to the kind of medical-surgical units from which they would have originated.

INITIAL EXPERIENCE

During the first 6 months of operation, from April through August of 1979, 40% of the patient rooms (or two of the five floors) were made available for patients during a period of active testing of the Cooperative Care concept in action. This was done because no other institution previously had experienced precisely this system of care delivery for inpatients. The nursing and educational staff needed time to feel comfortable with the physical separation from their patients for significant periods of time, and to see whether family members or friends could truly act responsibly as care partners. Physicians needed to gain experience in determining which of their patients could be managed more appropriately in this setting than in the types of more structured hospital units to which they were accustomed. Patients and families had to understand that their responsibilities were real, not superficial frills, and that the role of care partner was not just that of a glorified visitor.

A study of all patients admitted to Cooperative Care during the first 6 months of operation was done ("Quality Assurance Study," 1979) comparing them with patients with the same primary diagnosis admitted to the traditional medical-surgical nursing units during the preceding calendar year. Length of stay was higher by 3 days (19 vs. 16) for the patients transferred to Cooperative Care from traditional nursing units compared with patients with those primary diagnoses who underwent traditional care alone. However, length of stay for patients who were directly admitted to Cooperative Care was 40% shorter (4 vs. 7 days) compared with patients directly admitted to traditional medical-surgical nursing units for the same primary diagnoses.

The spectrum of diagnoses represented in Cooperative Care during this start up period was significantly different from that predicted prior to opening. The proportion of patients with cancer were, as expected, 20% of the admissions to the then newly opened Cooperative Care unit. The proportion with genitourinary diseases also was close at 11%, compared with the 10% predicted. But cardiovascular diseases accounted for a remarkable 44% of the patients admitted, rather than the paltry 16% expected. Hematological disorders, neurological disorders, and digestive diseases each accounted for 6%. All other diagnostic groups provided very small numbers of patients. Infectious disease, for example, was just over 1% of the early patient population.

Mean length of stay in the young Cooperative Care unit was 6.6 days, much shorter than the 10 days predicted.

THE EARLY YEARS

After the period of initial adjustment passed and Cooperative Care settled into a more routine mode of operation, a comparative study was undertaken, in conjunction with the School of Public Health of Johns Hopkins University (Chwalow et al, 1990). That study, which spanned the years 1981 through 1983, consisted of two distinct subgroups. The first subgroup was comprised of patients scheduled for direct admission to the medical center, who were randomly allocated to either Cooperative Care or traditional medical-surgical nursing units. The second subgroup consisted of patients on the surgical service in traditional hospital nursing units who were transferred to Cooperative Care for the latter part of their hospitalization, compared with a group who were not transferred. The two groups were matched for primary and secondary diagnoses and eligibility criteria for Cooperative Care. Of course, during this time the pattern of usage of Cooperative Care was still evolving. It continued to become more and more predominantly a site for direct admissions, like all other acute hospital units.

Analyzing the financial outcomes of the two subgroups (NYUMC evaluation, 1985) and looking at ancillary and routine departments and resource consumption, patients transferred to Cooperative Care were 15.3% less costly per day than non transferred patients, but they had a higher length of stay, so the savings per hospitalization were small, a mere 1.6 percent. The direct admission population, however, provided a dramatic cost savings. Their costs were 23.1% lower per day than traditional care, and with their lower mean length of stay the cost per hospitalization was down by a stunning 43%. If these numbers are combined in the ratio of the actual experience of direct admissions and transfers (using a ratio of 90% direct admissions to 10% transfers for this purpose), the overall savings in Cooperative Care would be 23% per day or 38% per hospitalization.

SUBSEQUENT EXPERIENCE

Over the next several years, the trends in utilization continued almost completely toward direct admissions, with few transfers. Average length of stay continued to drop, then leveled off at 4.5 days. More than 6 thousand patients entered each year. Mean age remained 55 years.

What about the flux backward from Cooperative Care to the traditional part of the hospital? Throughout these years, transfers out of Cooperative Care because of a change in clinical condition that led to an inability to maintain care in that setting occurred in only 8% of the patients, with well under 1% considered initially inappropriate and requiring transfer within the first 24 hours. The stability of these numbers as the case mix advanced over the years is testimony to the ability of Cooperative Care to provide safe and effective care for a wider variety of clinical problems of broader scope than that originally contemplated prior to its opening.

Over the years, the vast majority of patients in Cooperative Care have been on the medical service, which accounts for 80 to 85% of total admissions. Thus, it is quite understandable that the disease spectrum is that of a medical, rather than a surgical, unit. The three largest diagnostic groups have been infectious diseases, cancer, and cardiovascular disease, each of which accounts for approximately one-fifth of the total patient load.

The high proportion of infectious disease patients is quite at variance with the initial projections and the early experience. It reflects the explosion of people afflicted with the human immunodeficiency virus and its complications. These patients are some of the sickest in the entire medical center, and are acknowledged to be best handled in the Cooperative Care environment. The involvement of the care partner provides exceptional benefit to this group of patients, and because the care partner is often the also-infected lover, there is a tendency at times to alternate patient/care partner roles between the two people on succeeding admissions.

STAFFING RATIOS

With the active participation of family or friends, the effect of the professional staff is, in essence, multiplied. Therefore, staffing ratios are 40% lower in Cooperative Care than on similar units in the traditional hospital. This translates into cost savings of approximately one-third that of usual care.

None of this would be possible were it not for the involvement of family or friend care partners. Their usefulness would be limited were it not for the structured educational component which is so strongly built into the Cooperative Care program. Because that principle has remained unaltered from the planning period to the present, the working criteria for patient selection have been stable, although the patient mix has been sicker. The criteria for admission remain:

1. the patient must be sick enough to warrant acute care hospitalization;
2. the patient should be mobile enough for the care partner to be able to handle transfers, toileting, and other personal needs in the room, generally bringing the patient to the centralized core services for clinical assessments and treatments, educational sessions and meals;
3. the patient should be stable enough so that intensive care unit monitoring is needed only for relatively short periods of time; and
4. the patient should have a family member or friend who can carry out the functions of a care partner.

With these few limitations, any disease process is potentially suitable for management in Cooperative Care.

3

CARE PARTNER FUNCTIONS

Anthony J. Grieco, Kimberly S. Glassman,
Grace Phelan, and Shirley A. Garnett

It has been said that "good friends are an essential ingredient for good health" (Eisenberg, 1979, p. 552). This axiom is particularly true in Cooperative Care, where the one-on-one observation and assistance of a "significant other" is the most important ingredient distinguishing this form of care from that of a traditional hospital unit.

WHO IS THE CARE PARTNER?

A "care partner" is a family member or other individual who accompanies the patient during the hospitalization. The care partner acts as companion and advocate by living with the patient in a homelike room, providing assistance with physical tasks, and reporting observations and symptoms to the professional staff. This is not merely enhancing the role of "visitor," as that implies a passive individual who episodically appears during the course of a hospitalization. Rather, the family member or friend who is acting as a care partner is transformed into an active participant who assists the patient and learns the techniques and strategies necessary to support the patient both while in the hospital and after discharge to home.

The physical separation of the patient's living accommodations from the core clinical facilities would make the Cooperative Care experience seem a very isolated one for the patient, were it not for the presence of the care partner. As each room houses just one patient, while there the patient and care partner can behave much as though they were in their own home. By and large healthy, the care partner is usually a close family member who will be assisting the patient later on at home. Cooperative Care provides the opportunity for him or her to learn during the hospitalization how to support the patient in learning self-care techniques, or how to provide the necessary care at home, if the patient will be unable to do so.

Rather than having one sole family member identified to act as a care partner throughout the entire hospital stay, a sequence of people often fulfill this function. We have found that such a series of family members and friends can equally well provide support for the patient and each other during a lengthy hospitalization.

Although in general our admission requirement is for the 24–hour presence of a care partner, shifts of individuals can be just as effective in assisting the patient. Less disruption of the family unit occurs with this system, as no one individual needs to miss work and other family responsibilities for a prolonged period of time. In addition, rotating the responsibility for being a care partner generates a broader network of support for after discharge.

Following an invasive procedure, most patients are taken to the Observation Unit for temporary care. This is a six-bed area which functions much like a recovery room, with staff in constant attendance. Here, not only is the care provided by the staff, but under the guidance of registered nurses and nursing attendants the care partner learns what to observe about the patient and report to the professionals later when patient and partner are back in their own room. As a result, patients who have undergone invasive procedures, such as coronary angiography, bronchoscopy, or liver biopsy, quickly become aware of the expected "normal" and potential "abnormal" responses to the procedure and treatment, and learn first-hand what observations the patient/care partner team should make. In the process, they become more comfortable dealing with this situation.

Some patients may be placed on limited activity for the evening following a procedure. The care partner then acts as a reporter and messenger, as well as a companion and observer. He/she obtains snacks and supplies and assists the patient with meals, toileting, and so

forth—tasks very similar to what may be required of them at home under similar circumstances.

Technical procedures, such as intravenous infusions of antibiotics or
chemotherapy, blood and platelet transfusions, and specialized treatments are administered in the therapeutic center, by and under the supervision of professional nurses. If these treatments are required at
home, the patient/care partner team is scheduled to attend educational classes together so that they will better learn how to do their
part of these tasks properly. They will then perform them in conjunction with the professionals while in Cooperative Care, so that they will
be more proficient in these tasks by the time of discharge.

WHAT ARE THE RESPONSIBILITIES OF THE CARE PARTNER?

Let's look at some of the specific tasks and responsibilities which the
care partner is charged with carrying out. The major ones are:

1) providing physical assistance in the room;
2) providing emotional support for the patient;
3) making observations;
4) participating in the treatment regimen;
5) calling for assistance; and
6) performing personal chores.

It would be helpful at this point to examine these responsibilities one-
by-one in a little detail.

Providing Physical Assistance

Since there are no nurses or nurse-aides in the patient rooms, any routine physical assistance the patient needs is provided by the care partner. By and large, this is a task for which the family member or friend
is very well suited, since it is a function which people provide regularly for one another in the home. Of course, with the diminished capability of the patient during an acute illness, the needs are likely to
be greater than when the patient is well. Consequently, some steps
must be taken to avoid having this situation evolve into an excessive
strain for the care partner.

For example, if the patient needs assistance in transferring to and
from bed, the care partner must be physically able to provide the
needed help. He or she may need direct instruction in the proper tech-

nique from the nursing staff. Similarly, wheelchair safety is a commonly needed instruction, so frequently needed that it is handled in part by a closed-circuit television program. Likewise, a physical therapist might be enlisted to help teach both the patient and the care partner the proper way to use a cane or walker, and how to supervise the patient using such an assistive device. Simply supporting a patient with unsteady gait is no easy trick for the uninitiated, and this also would require evaluation and teaching by the educational and clinical staff.

Personal hygiene and other activities of daily living may be inadequate without the help of the care partner in washing and toileting, as well as feeding and dressing. Teaching the family the tricks which will make these tasks easier to accomplish goes a long way in making the adjustment to longer-term care at home more tolerable.

A major care partner responsibility under the broad topic of physical assistance is protection from falls. Our studies demonstrate a 40% reduction in falls by patients in Cooperative Care compared with a matched group on traditional medical-surgical nursing units. This is accomplished mostly by the constant attention and presence of the care partner, alertly on the scene doing what comes naturally to protect a loved one who appears unsteady.

Wandering by confused patients is a worry in most traditional hospital units. It often leads to physical restraints, which themselves bring significant hazards, such as decubitus ulcers, aspiration and physical injury. In Cooperative Care, wandering is prevented by the presence of the family member or friend. This is a very effective method of maintaining orientation to place, and certainly much more practical and useful than oversedation or the use of side-rails and restraints. The quiet and lack of confusing distractions in the patient room is another help in this regard, since the noisy hospital apparatus and personnel are located at great distance from the patient rooms, on a different floor entirely.

Physically helping a patient at mealtime is another function which is better performed by a care partner than by the hospital staff. Certainly this is a homelike and natural task, and a family member or close friend who is loving and kind can do it with affection, using both the verbal and nonverbal communications which only families appear to understand. Of course, the family member also does not have the time pressure of the responsibility for many other patients as is the case with the nurses or nurse-aides on a traditional unit, so there is less hurrying and more persistence with feeding a slow, obstreperous patient.

Ensuring adequate fluid intake, and accurately recording intake of food and liquid and output of urine and stool, can be more compulsively accomplished by care partners than by hospital staff. Because care partners are constantly with the patient, they give this responsibility a high priority on their list of daily assignments.

Assistance with bathing is a bit trickier. Although the care partner generally is capable of accomplishing washing and bathing for the patient, Cooperative Care room assignments need to be made keeping in mind whether a wheelchair-accessible shower stall is needed rather than a bathroom with a full bathtub.

Urinary and bowel function is another challenge faced by the care partner. Helping the patient on and off the toilet, and avoiding incontinence of urine and stool, although difficult and wearing at times, is actually better accomplished by the everpresent care partner than by the sometimes slow-to-respond hospital staff, who may not realize that a quick response to the call-bell might obviate the need to change soiled bedclothes and sheets.

Providing Emotional Support

The presence of a family member or close friend has obvious benefits in emotionally supporting the acutely or chronically ill patient. Loneliness is avoided, depression and dejection are at least faced openly, and the fear of unpleasant or painful treatments can be assuaged by hand holding and compassion.

But this is not a one-way street. The care partner benefits emotionally as well. There is no worrying about what is happening to the patient in the hospital while the family is at home. There is no problem with travelling back and forth, not being sure of being on the scene when the patient is in need of solace.

In Cooperative Care, it is quite common for patients to try to look their best in order to please the care partner. Patients are more likely to dress in street clothing rather than in pajamas, and they spend more time up in chairs and walking than their counterparts on medical-surgical units. Patients often make obvious attempts to help care partners with their own needs for consolation and reassurance.

Care partners also fill a role as entertainers for the patients, whether it be by talking, reading, watching television, playing cards, or doing other homelike activities. There is frequently an overt attempt to make the hospitalization for a serious illness appear superficially more like a leisure cruise than an institutional confinement. This "game" is so frequently seen by our staff that they accept it as a natural and beneficial consequence of the Cooperative Care environment. Of course, when children are sick, "playing" helps them to cope with their anxieties. Cooperative Care demonstrates that the same is true with many adults.

Making Observations

Perhaps the most important technical task performed by a care partner is making observations about the patient's condition. The talents and skills which a family member or friend needs in order to function at a high level of competence in making accurate clinical observations can be divided into two categories: 1) personal knowledge of the patient's range of normal behaviors and appearance, and 2) understanding of the disease process and its possible manifestations.

As far as the first category is concerned, in many instances family and friends are much better equipped to recognize significant subtleties in appearance of a loved one than are professionals, who have not seen the patient before and need to rely entirely upon their clinical acumen. The second category needs to be addressed by education of the care partner. Because the care partner has the advantage of personal knowledge, and because of the love and concern and devotion they have for the patient, accomplishing the needed learning about the disease process generally is not difficult in the Cooperative Care setting, particularly because there is ample opportunity for repeated reinforcement and review by the professional staff.

For example, the care partner is more likely to first notice slight changes in the patient's thinking, speech pattern or behavior. By contrast, it is much simpler to teach people how to find and count the pulse, or how to look for signs of bleeding or weakness, than it is to teach someone how to make those more significant observations for which the care partner is ideally equipped.

Participating In The Treatment Regimen

By enlisting the care partner's assistance in carrying out the treatment regimen, medication administration is greatly facilitated. Following instruction by a pharmacist or nurse-educator, and review by a nurse-clinician, the patient/care partner team may be given responsibility for administering all oral medications. Certainly this reduces the nursing workload. More importantly, it improves patient safety by drastically limiting the potential for medication administration errors. This is so because the patient/care partner team have only one patient to deal with, so they cannot inadvertently give the drugs to the wrong person. The team almost always treats medication with great respect, particularly because the aura of most hospitals forbids their collaboration in this venture, and they appear eager to earn the nurse's trust.

Watching, then doing it together, then doing it with the nurse observing, then doing it alone in the room, are the stages of development in a care partner's responsibility for changing dressings or dealing with appliances, devices, and equipment, such as inhalation therapy. Similarly, insulin administration is better taught in the empowering Cooperative Care setting than in the usual hospital environment, which denigrates patient independence as a safety hazard.

Selecting food from the cafeteria-style dining room is another aspect of the therapeutic regimen, which is a thrice-daily learning opportunity in Cooperative Care.

Calling For Assistance

If the care partner did nothing else but be available to call for assistance in the event it were urgently needed, his or her presence would be justified. The safety feature that makes Cooperative Care work as an acute care hospital unit is that someone is constantly present to observe and to call for assistance. Traditional hospital units accomplish this by keeping the patient's room door open so that passing staff can peek in to see whether anything untoward is happening, but that is only episodic observation. Cooperative Care has continuous observation by the care partner, so the call for assistance comes earlier than in most medical-surgical nursing units.

The power of this feature of Cooperative Care should not be underestimated. Given instruction as to what should be expected, and the personal insights possessed by a close family member it is not at all surprising that emergency calls to the Therapeutic Center trigger an immediate response. Usually, a nurse-clinician is dispatched to the room to assess the situation firsthand. An emergency-response team might follow, if it appears warranted. The patient might need stabilization in the room, or might need to be transferred to the observation unit for closer bedside nursing attention and more intensive care.

Performing Personal Chores

With both the patient and "significant other" in the hospital together, personal chores at home need attention as well. The care partner might therefore need to have some time off to go back and forth to handle these details. This gives some respite, and usually can be arranged for times during which the patient's safety would not be an issue, such as times when the professional staff are directly observing or treating the patient.

CARE PARTNER STRESS AND COPING

Faced with all these responsibilities, how does the care partner cope? In order to answer that question for a specific individual, it is helpful first to look at the roles which the patient and care partner team have performed prior to the hospitalization. For example, who has generally provided the family strength over the years, the patient or the care partner? Has the care partner ever been in the position of requiring care from the person who is now the patient? Are other family members or friends available to be called upon for additional help if it becomes needed during this hospitalization? Are there major stresses, other than the illness itself, which need to be faced concurrently? How have the patient and care partner handled stresses in the past?

In helping the care partner to cope, the first step is to recognize and acknowledge that he or she has emotional needs which must be addressed and met. One way to start this process is to enable the care partner to verbalize his or her frustrations, since simply having the opportunity to vent and to obtain positive reinforcement may suffice as a compensation vehicle.

In analyzing the stresses which care partners might undergo, we should look at the common complaints that family members express when they care for patients at home (Robinson, 1983). They talk of interrupted sleep, inconvenience, excessive physical demands, restricted free time, limited social life, disrupted family routine, and sacrifice of personal needs. To overcome these complaints, home care partners need time for recreation, privacy and relaxation. The annoyances that care partners face in Cooperative Care are not dissimilar, and the solutions are comparable.

If the patient and care partner are amenable, adjustment to the care partner role is easily accomplished. But if arguments ensue, or if the patient is very confused or agitated, then it can be predicted that the care partner will have a more difficult time adjusting to the role. In other words, the burden faced by a care partner in dealing with the patient's physical disability is less of a trial than is dealing with the patient's intellectual or emotional disability (Poulshock & Deimling, 1984).

In the home, a major challenge which the family often finds overwhelming is dealing with a patient's urinary or fecal incontinence. In

Cooperative Care, this task is handled by the staff. If it becomes a persistent problem, it might lead to transfer of the patient to the more traditional area of the hospital.

When there has been a prolonged or complicated hospitalization, particularly in instances in which the patient has been in the Intensive Care Unit before transfer to Cooperative Care, the staff needs to look for the possibility of "burnout" on the part of the care partner. In some cases, care partners are able to verbalize their feelings; in other cases, the signs might be more subtle, such as the care partner being terse in interactions with the patient or the staff. The care partner might be reluctant to admit his or her exhaustion, in part because the patient appears so sick and the care partner feels the responsibility to be of help.

Overall, when there is a partnership of caring among the patient, the family and the staff, with emotional support and positive feedback flowing from all three sources, the care partner arrangement works well. But when the relationship deteriorates into that of a totally dominant caretaker and a completely passive receiver of care, the stress level for the care partner is apt to rise to the point of disintegrating the partnership role and making continued stay in Cooperative Care tenuous. An astute nurse or social worker might detect this progression, which is particularly dangerous when the care partner harbors resentment but is reluctant to discuss these feelings. The staff is taught to use every opportunity to problem-solve with the patient and the care partner as to what alternatives are available. For example: Can other family members or friends alternate the caring responsibility? Can the care partner leave the unit for the period of time in which the patient is receiving treatment from the nurses, or when the patient is off for tests? It might be determined that the patient would be safe when the care partner is not on site. Or, a hired care partner may be urgently needed, to provide a respite to tide the family member over the crisis.

How else can the family be helped to cope? The care partner will be able to cope more effectively if he or she can be assisted in achieving the following levels of functional competence:

1. feeling self-reliant in handling the patient's physical needs in the room;
2. feeling confident about their grasp of the disease process and the therapeutic regimen;
3. knowing how to maintain the patient's personal hygiene;
4. gaining a sense of accomplishment and increased self-esteem about their role in helping the patient;

5. having the emotional stability to deal with their responsibilities;
6. being a participant in reaching decisions about care; and
7. accepting proffered help and direction toward available resources (Choi, Josten, & Christensen, 1983).

Care partner support groups offer the opportunity to discuss common concerns, as well as give the staff the occasion to assess their coping mechanisms. In unusual circumstances, the strain on the care partner leads to transfer of the patient to the more traditional part of the hospital.

CARE PARTNER AVAILABILITY

Questions that are frequently asked in regard to care partners are: "Are they capable?" and "Do they really agree to stay?" The answer to the first question is an overwhelmingly resounding "Yes!" As discussed above, this is not surprising, since the role of the care partner at Cooperative Care is not much different from the role a family member would play at home before admission or after discharge. The care partner is not eager to assume the role of the health care professional, but is fully capable of helping with activities of daily living, reporting observations to the professional staff, and providing the patient with companionship and support. They also are eager to become more knowledgeable about what they will need to do at home, including when to call the physician, what the patient should eat, or how to administer total parenteral nutrition. The care partner becomes a great asset to the patient and to the professionals. How different this is from the traditional setting, in which visitors and staff sometimes assume an almost adversarial role. The visitors who "stay too long" or "ask too many questions" or insist on doing tasks for the patient a certain way because they have been doing it at home that way are sometimes seen as hindrances. In Cooperative Care, these are almost nonexistent problems; the staff recognizes and appreciates the abilities of the care partner.

The second question, "Do they really agree to stay?" is more complicated. In modern times, with the economic need for all members of a family to work, with families smaller in size than in past generations, and with offspring often in widely scattered geographic locations, it may be challenging to locate a family member who is available to serve as a care partner. However, since the hospitalizations tend to be short, averaging 4 or 5 days, this is not an insurmountable problem for most families. Rather than focussing entirely upon a spouse, daughter, or son, a wider circle of friends and relatives may need to be scanned for possible care partners. Rotating the responsibility among that larger group of people may solve the issue of availability more neatly.

Although the prototypical caring family member at home is a woman (Crossman, London, & Barry, 1981), especially a spouse or daughter, in Cooperative Care, particularly for patients who have acquired immunodeficiency syndrome, young men caring for other young men is quite frequently seen, and the experience tends to be extraordinarily successful.

At the time of admission to Cooperative Care, the availability and abilities of the care partner are assessed by the nurse-educator and the nurse-clinician. Questions asked include: Will the "team" be safe in the room together? How have they been managing at home? Is the care partner physically capable of assisting with any needed activities of daily living? In addition, the patient/care partner team are assessed in terms of their understanding. For example, is this a new diagnosis? Do they know when to contact the nurse? Their emotional adjustment also is assessed. How do they interact? Who does the talking? All of this is helpful, not only in assessing the pair, but also in developing the plan of care.

Care partners, themselves, are not always free of illness. In fact, sometimes Cooperative Care is a better option than is a traditional hospital unit. Because the currently acutely ill patient is, over the long term, the healthier one of the pair, and he/she feels much more secure in having the chronically ill care partner nearby so that the safety of that person can be assured. That emotion—of feeling responsible for the well-being of a loved one—is precisely the reason that care partners in Cooperative Care work so well. That combined sense of love and responsibility is the secret behind the success of Cooperative Care. Without it the unit would not be able to exist.

4

THE PATIENT'S PERSPECTIVE

Margaret L. McClure and Wanda Kowalski

This chapter looks at caring in the Cooperative Care environment from the patient's perspective. This is a very important concept, especially since caring is central to the Cooperative Care philosophy.

Among the interesting things about the word "care" are the varied and disparate connotations that can be implied from its use. On the one hand, used as a noun, the meaning can be rather negative. In fact, one dictionary defines care as "a suffering of mind." A care, then, is generally an unwanted burden or worry. As an intransitive verb, however, caring generally takes on a much more positive connotation, filled with a sense of warmth, nurturing, and compassion. Professional caring, of course, goes beyond the interpersonal sphere and encompasses the added dimension of technical competence.

What we are going to attempt to describe for you is what it is to care, to deliver care, and to receive care in this rather unique environment. In order to do that, we have interviewed a number of patients, care partners, and staff members so that the reader may have the advantage of their perspectives and, in some cases, hear their own words. It should be added that this was a surprisingly exciting opportunity for us to learn a great deal more and to develop new insights into the Cooperative Care experience.

The patients who were kind enough to talk about Cooperative Care represented a diverse group, both in terms of diagnoses and age. Several had been in Cooperative Care previously; in fact one gentleman indicated that during his last visit his wife had been the patient and he the care partner. One characteristic that they shared: all were quite ill, and most with chronic illnesses that would require continuing treatment beyond the hospital; these were not transitional care patients.

Cooperative Care is a unit in which we share the provision of care with patients and their care partners. There are a number of characteristics that the individuals who were a part of this environment discussed during our conversations. Without question, one of the most important characteristics concerned the area of control. Either explicitly or implicitly, this factor was mentioned by virtually everyone, and was generally viewed as having a positive impact on the quality of patient life. Seen from one point of view, it can be said that a substantial amount of responsibility and control are shifted to the patient and his or her care partner, and this is certainly true for those who are transferred to Cooperative Care from the traditional part of the hospital. However, for those who are directly admitted to Cooperative Care, it is more accurate to say that principal control and responsibility are retained by patients, not forfeited as they are in the usual hospital situation.

FREEDOM

Control was described as having several subsets, the first of which is freedom. By this is meant freedom of movement and of decision making; in other words, a real sense of independence. Patients in particular value the fact that they are not totally dependent on others, especially strangers, for the "little things" that constitute the bulk of their activities. Having the right to decide when to eat, go to bed, get up, etc., sounds fairly mundane and unimportant; yet viewed through the eyes of the patient, these activities do take on a different light. This was brought home rather sharply by one elderly lady who is wheelchair-bound. In a traditional setting, she would be forced to get out of bed and go back to bed, generally at the convenience of the nursing staff, even the most caring of whom often find themselves too harried to respond to folks like this on an individualized basis.

More interesting were the insightful (and touching) comments concerning the control/freedom aspects that were made by two different patients, both of whom had serious diagnoses. They alluded to the fact that being independent and less helpless made them feel hopeful. This, they believe, was conducive to their getting well and going home sooner. One AIDS patient even said that he believed that this psychological mindset had extended his life.

When staff describe this phenomenon, they indicate that one of the benefits of the patients' independent orientation is that it makes them more willing participants in their own care. For example, one of the social workers observed that patients in traditional hospital settings have often become so psychologically dependent that it is difficult for them to provide input into their own discharge plans.

The nursing staff particularly pointed out that freedom to participate more freely in making decisions, especially the decision to wear street clothes, allows patients to maintain their own identity. The famous sociologist Talcott Parsons (1951) wrote extensively about the ways in which people who are ill assume what he termed the "sick" role. He described a kind of learned helplessness that develops and serves to rob the individual of his self-identity as a fully functioning person, in charge of his own destiny.

In reviewing these comments related to freedom, it seems clear that the Cooperative Care environment acts to overcome some of the negative aspects of the sick role for the patients who are there, despite the fact that many have dreadful, even overwhelming, health problems.

The only negative comments that were made regarding the freedom of patients were made by some of the professionals. As one might expect, these criticisms were related entirely to the fact that patients and their care partners are sometimes hard to locate. They are not always where the professionals might want them to be and when they want them to be there.

PRIVACY/QUIET

A second component of control is that of privacy and quiet. This was particularly noted by the patients, although some of the professionals mentioned it as well. Very often, patients specifically noted that their rooms on the patient floors were peaceful and restful; certainly not an observation likely to be made concerning the traditional medical/surgical unit! One woman, whose cardiac condition has necessitated multiple admissions in both areas, spoke very positively about the lack of a stranger as a roommate, indicating that too often she had been with other patients whose clinical conditions or personal habits had been disturbing to her in one way or another. Further, she cited the inevitable problems in traditional hospital units with visitors, whose presence more often than not is an annoyance to a roommate. On the other hand, entertaining children or grandchildren, including sharing meals with them, is easier in the Cooperative Care environment.

It was interesting that in various ways patients talked about the extent to which the presence of a care partner decreased their loneliness during hospitalization. Without explicitly saying so, patients made a clear implication that loneliness is a problem in the traditional hospital; this is probably the consummate example of the lonely-in-a-crowd syndrome.

Professionals, for their part, reported that patients experienced some loneliness or insecurity during the hours when their care partners are not present. The nurses say that patients sometimes handle this by coming to them with questions to which they already know the answers, or with other requests for assistance that are actually excuses for contact. In other instances, they may walk down the hallway in front of the nurses exam rooms and wave, "just to say hello," and verify that the nurse is still there for them.

EDUCATION

An additional characteristic that is fundamental to the entire Cooperative Care approach is that of education. This represents yet another way in which patients and care partners achieve control. As one person said, "We feel more in control because we know what's going on, what to expect." This feature is especially appreciated by care partners because they learn how they can cope, what they can contribute and even how to take effective charge if it becomes necessary. In the words of one:

> The nurses explain to me as her caregiver how I can handle her better and I think that's the most wonderful thing in the world. I'm not a novice now. . . . And they're always there to guide you. It isn't that they're just there to take care of her. They enlighten me also so that I can take care of her after she leaves here.

The professionals share this point of view. As one of the social workers said, "People definitely leave here better prepared to cope." In addition, the staff perceive that the patients are less anxious in Cooperative Care, because information is shared so freely.

DECREASED FEAR

One surprising characteristic mentioned by virtually all of the patients and care partners was the extent to which the Cooperative Care environment reduced their fears and the fears of others. On closer examination, it becomes evident that the increased sense of control acts to reduce the feeling of vulnerability.

An AIDS patient, who has had repeated admissions, stated that he no longer becomes anxious when he has to be admitted, despite the fact that this represents a setback for him. He sees this as a sharp contrast to the experience of others in similar circumstances who are admitted to traditional settings.

This decrease in fear is attributed by many to the total environment. For example, one care partner who had several hospitalizations elsewhere said, "I can tell now the patients who come in here when it is the first day and the second day and I can see such a change in everyone's attitude. You know, the fear and heartbreak in their face and eyes at first and then the slow development of hope." And a patient said, "No matter how sick you feel, you don't feel scared; you don't feel that at all."

Some patients commented that they look upon their rooms almost as retreats, because no treatments take place there. It occurred to us that we follow a longstanding principle in pediatric nursing [holds] that, to the extent possible, we try not to do any painful procedures for children in their cribs. Rather, we take them to a central treatment room, so that the crib becomes a place they can identify with safety and security. Perhaps we have missed the boat with adults in this regard. Perhaps, like children, everyone needs a safe place that they can make their own, where they are in control. This may be one of the unplanned, unexpected consequences of the Cooperative Care environment.

The nursing staff added a further thought: that the presence of care partners also reduces the stress for patients because they sense that they have an advocate with them, and this, in turn, reduces their vulnerability.

RESPONSIBILITY

Along with the control comes, for the patient and care partner, added responsibility. This area tended to be discussed mostly by the staff. One issue that they raised in this regard was the need for orientation on the part of all concerned. The occasional patient is not anxious to

maintain a self-care mode. One example was the diabetic who indicated he would prefer that the nurses take over monitoring his glucose
levels and administering his insulin, despite the fact that he did this
for himself at home. Needless to say, it takes a fair amount of work on
the part of the staff to make this person feel well-supported and cared
for; sometimes compromises have to be made to insure that patients do
not feel short-changed.

Interestingly enough, the Cooperative Care approach also requires a
great deal of adjustment on the part of the professional staff. This is
particularly true for the nurses, who are accustomed to monitoring inpatients much more closely, and who sense a great loss of control when
they begin to practice in Cooperative Care. This is probably best
summed up by the nurse who said: "Loss of control was the biggest
thing for me when I came here. I worked in the ICU where I controlled
everything—the blood pressure, the urine output—you name it, we had
a dial for it."

For nurses, one of the big concerns is that patients exercise their responsibility reliably. They put a great deal of effort into ensuring that
patients and care partners are safe and coping well when they are
away from the staff's watchful eyes.

THE CARE PARTNER

Key to the success of Cooperative Care is the involvement of a care
partner. It should be remembered that Cooperative Care was not conceived as a cost-saving delivery system, but rather as a means by
which to improve the quality of patient care. The assumption of care
partner participation was that caring is often best done by someone
who has a longstanding caring relationship with the patient—borrow-
ing from the jargon of the social sciences, a "significant other."

We often speak of the care partner as a single individual. This may
be misleading; for while there is only one designated care partner at
any given time, some patients have several different people who take
turns doing the job and the particular individual may or may not be a
member of the individual's household.

The Patient's Point Of View

From the patient's point of view, the care partner is clearly a welcome
resource, and patients are very happy not to have to send them away
at a particular time because visiting hours are over. They describe the
care partner as "someone who understands you and everything you

need," saying, again, that their presence dispels the loneliness of a regular hospital.

In response to the question "How do you think your care partner feels about being here?" one woman said that her husband (who is retired) used to come and stay all day when she was in the main hospital, so he is much more comfortable and at ease in the Cooperative Care setting.

Another, more insightful, statement came from a young man who said, "My care partner is my father. He lives in California and in a bizarre way, I'm almost glad I needed him this time because we don't get to see each other often. So we've been together for two weeks and in a way, it has been wonderful." It may be, then, that having a care partner creates opportunities to re create or even repair relationships.

The only negative comment made by patients in this area was said jokingly by an older gentleman, who indicated that his wife takes "too much care of me."

The Care Partner Point Of View

For the most part, care partners welcomed the opportunity to be with the patient. As one patient's wife said, "I feel like we are facing it (the illness) together and this helps us both. It saves the wear and tear of being left out and being worried at home." This setting, then, provides a kind of mutual support, a feature that almost everyone involved in the unit corroborates.

Two highly respected nursing scholars recently published a text entitled *The Primacy of Caring* (Benner & Wrubel, 1989). One of their major themes concerns the idea that healing efforts are more efficacious in a caring context. They would have been pleased to see their ideas supported by the care partners in Cooperative Care. In fact, one woman stated that she believed that just her very presence was helping her husband to heal.

There are negative aspects to the care partner role, particularly if the patient needs someone around the clock. Many care partners have other responsibilities, such as work or child care, and find it difficult to rearrange their lives to accommodate the patient's needs. In other instances, care partners experience the responsibility as stressful and exhausting, especially if they are unable to take a break.

The staff also have observed and been subject to some hostility on the part of a few care partners, when the patients require a great deal of bedside care and they perceive that the staff "should" be doing this work. Our impression is that this attitude probably develops among care partners who are not members of the patient's immediate family or household.

THE PROFESSIONAL'S POINT OF VIEW

The professionals in Cooperative Care find that the presence of a care partner both enables their work and helps them to better care for the patients because they get a fuller picture of the patient's life outside the hospital. As one staff member pointed out, in traditional settings it is easy to forget that the patient comes from a community to which he will return. In Cooperative Care the professionals feel more pressure to adapt to patients and their individualized needs.

The availability of family is particularly appreciated when teaching and discharge planning are taking place. The staff sense that the changes necessary to accommodate the patient are more likely to be understood and incorporated when the patient is supported by someone who has been part of the experience. As an example, one nutritionist pointed to the benefit of having a care partner, who may be the person who purchases and/or prepares the food at home, incorporated into her counselling sessions.

Another plus is the care partner's role in monitoring patients. Apparently most are absolutely meticulous in their observations, reporting very reliably the information that the nurse, nutritionist or pharmacist might require.

Care partners are a concern to the professional staff as well. There are several reasons for this. First, as discussed earlier, some can become overtired and even burned out from the physical and, perhaps more important, psychological demands of the role. The nurses indicated that they must be attuned to this problem and stated that they often have to intervene, convincing a care partner to get relief when it seems indicated.

The staff are aware that there are probably tensions between patients and care partners. People who are sick often have a great deal of understandable anger concerning their conditions. In traditional settings, the family may have some of this displaced onto them; quite often, however, the staff help to absorb some as well, because of the limited family contact. In Cooperative Care, the continuous interaction between patients and care partners provides more opportunities for the family to bear the brunt of this anger. Clearly all of us feel safer acting out with those closest to us, rather than with strangers, and there is even more risk involved in venting when the object of your ire is your health care provider. Thus, there is a syndrome that takes place which was once described in a song, "You always hurt the one you love." This problem can obviously become more difficult when the care partner is not in a position to get away.

The issue of fatigue and burnout of significant others is one that all of us in health care will have to confront in a more systematic and meaningful way in the future. Concern for the toll that is taken when one is caring for loved ones has been receiving increasing concern as we move further into the sicker-quicker era. There is a cost that is paid by the caregiver, sometimes a high cost, that has the potential to become a societal cost. We need to devise more and better support systems for these individuals.

PATIENT COMMUNITY

In observing the daily routine in Cooperative Care, it becomes immediately apparent that the patients and care partners often develop a sense of community which in some respects can be likened to a subculture. This is, of course, a side effect of the multiple opportunities for group situations. For example, activities such as congregate dining, education center classes, and happy hour all lend themselves to the development of more relationships between and among the participants.

Almost everyone who described Cooperative Care mentioned the mutual support that this sense of community engenders. Not only is there socializing that provides for diversion, there is also a real interest in helping each other and in sharing problems and solutions. Thus, while patients and care partners are not forced to spend time with each other, as they are with roommates in traditional settings, they are able to seek each other out when they feel the need for companionship or assistance.

One elderly woman reported seeing a young girl who was being admitted and noted that she looked frightened. She said something encouraging and gave her a hug. The next evening the girl arrived at the woman's door with a bouquet of flowers saying, "You can't imagine what that hug meant to me!"

There are, of course, negative aspects to such increased exposure to other patients. Some people simply do not like to be around sick people, even if they themselves are sick. It would be difficult, if not impossible, to shield oneself from other patients in Cooperative Care.

One other negative feature was mentioned by a nutritionist. She said that on occasion the formal classes have to compete with the informal groups where information is shared. She added that this is especially problematic if there are people there who have become enamored of some of the fads and quackery that occasionally catch the lay public's attention and enthusiasm.

THE NEW PATIENT

Patients and family who are new to the Cooperative Care environment are easy to identify. They combine the anxious look of a patient with a medical problem and the confused appearance of someone checking into a strange hotel. Clutching their suitcases, they appear overwhelmed and uncomfortable with this unorthodox method of care delivery. "Where will I sleep?" "How will I get my meals?" "How will you find me if you need me?" "How will I get you?" "Are you sure this is a *real* hospital?"

First impressions are important, and ancillary personnel play a vital role in assuring the patient they will be well cared for. Clerks who project a calm, professional manner and housekeeping staff who smile and say "Of course, we have patients like you all the time" have worked miracles in calming newcomers.

Once given the keys to their room, a tangible symbol of their independent role, patients seem to stand a little straighter. Patients and care partners defer to each other as to who will hold the keys; jokes are exchanged regarding the need for identification tags for patients as well as staff and the integration into the culture of Cooperative Care begins.

The orientation film which is shown immediately upon admission has proven invaluable in answering many of the patients' questions about the daily operations of the unit. In the past, patients who entered the unit at an hour too late to view the orientation film were markedly less comfortable, and made many more phone calls to the central nursing station than did patients who viewed the film. This observation of the orientation film's capacity for reassurance resulted in its being one of the first items to go on the closed circuit television channel.

Patients appear to be most concerned about how their doctor will find them, how other professional staff will find them, and how they will find their meals. After a visit with the primary physician, proving that one could indeed be found in this strange, new environment, they begin to accept the concept of Cooperative Care as a "real hospital" even more readily. The meeting with their nurse and the provision of a schedule of appointments; the discussion and/or initiation of self-administration of medication; and the reinforcement of how to summon help in an emergency only serve to bolster the patient's self-confidence.

The forced socialization of the dining room also aids in adaptation to the new environment. Sitting through a meal with a more seasoned patient and care partner provides many helpful "how-tos" to the rookie patient. They also provide living proof that Cooperative Care can and does work. Many former Cooperative Care patients can bear witness to the swift, effective intervention of the professional staff in cases of hypoglycemia, seizures, cardiac arrhythmias, and even cardiac arrest.

The mealtime experience also encourages patients to, once again, perceive themselves as active participants in their own care. Walking to a dining room, dressed in one's own clothes, and making choices about what one will or will not eat are adult behaviors that reinforce the message of patient control. Professional staff realized how successful they had been at returning control to the patient when the very same individuals who worried that their doctor would never find them began refusing to interrupt their meals for contacts with the professional staff.

ADMINISTRATIVE ASPECTS

It was interesting to note how many patients talked about some of the administrative aspects of Cooperative Care. In particular, all seemed to be aware of the decreased costs associated with delivering care in this setting. They spoke about this in a very positive way. As one individual said, "It makes so much sense." They understood that there was less need for large numbers of staff and that the physical facility itself was less expensive.

In particular, many discussed the fact that the staff is better utilized. They perceived that the professionals are not bogged down by menial tasks and that they are therefore better able to concentrate on the kinds of things that best use their knowledge. One individual said that he believed that the nurses in Cooperative Care were so positive because they are certain that what they are doing really matters. Another talked about the amount of knowledge that the nursing staff demonstrates when they are teaching, as they do whenever he interacts with them. From their perspective, the staff discussed the need for experienced practitioners to work in Cooperative Care because of the heavy teaching/counselling role and the independent nature of their practice.

The reader will probably be interested to learn that the patients frequently spoke of the need for other hospitals to develop Cooperative Care units. In fact, an AIDS patient who will probably be forced to relocate in the near future, stated that he hated the thought of leaving New York City because he knew that he would not find another Cooperative Care in his new location.

PROFESSIONAL PRACTICE CLIMATE

Almost since its inception, we have been aware of the fact that the staff members in Cooperative Care find the environment highly satisfying for their practice. They frequently talk about their ability to develop important and meaningful relationships with their patients. They have a sense that they truly make a difference and have an important impact on patients during the course of their admission and, indeed, long after they are discharged home.

Many report that Cooperative Care fosters much more of an interdisciplinary approach, not only through the formal team meetings that are held regularly, but also through the ongoing informal interactions that take place during the course of any given day. In addition, like the patients, the professional staff believe that their time is spent focused primarily on the kinds of work that utilize their knowledge and skills fully. As a nutritionist stated, "Finally, time has been designated for me to teach the patient." She went on to indicate that she is able to do this not only because it is an expectation in the setting, but also because she can rely on the care partner and the patient to take care of collecting and reporting data related to calorie counts, how the patient is tolerating supplemental feeding, etc. In addition, across all disciplines, professionals feel the sense of autonomy in relation to their practice.

In a recent study (Valentine, 1989), patients and professionals participated in an examination of the concept of caring. Patients rated the following components as most important:

1) being knowledgeable about the illness;
2) having flexibility to determine needs and respond to them;
3) teaching patients to meet their own needs as much as possible; and
4) giving the patient a way to have control.

Perhaps it is safe to conclude that the success we have had in Cooperative Care for the past 15 years is really based on the fact that it so closely meets the patients' definition of caring.

5

THE FAMILY'S PERSPECTIVE

Salvador Minuchin and Patricia Minuchin

Traditional medicine has always searched for the magic bullet: the one-to-one correlation of cure to illness. Though modern medicine has gained an understanding of the more complex biopsychosocial nature of health and illness, it is still characterized by an individual focus, and by the lingering hope of finding the correct match between biology and pharmacology.

The architectural design of most hospital wards, written, as it were, in concrete, carries the medical assumption that a sick person must be separated from his or her usual social context, "garaged" in the hospital where the illness will be treated, and then returned to his or her significant people. In one new building of a New York City hospital, the psychiatric ward was built with such an economy of space that a child in crisis had to be separated from family members. The space for interview and examination allowed only for the medical team and the child. It was clear for the architect that the child was the container of the illness. The family's function was to provide information, and to wait.

The Cooperative Care Center at New York University Medical Center is a notable exception to this prevailing framework for hospital life. By including the care partner, the unit implicitly hospitalizes part of the family, thus organizing a completely different type of hospital experience for the patient. Also inherent in the architecture is a demand for a new conceptualization of illness and cure—a challenge to the biological model of medicine, and the opening up of possibilities for a true family medicine to be practiced in the hospital setting.

THE FAMILY IN COOPERATIVE CARE

In the 1980s, the authors came to the Cooperative Care unit to interview patients, their care partners, and families about the experience of illness. We had been impressed by the structure of the unit, with its evident understanding of human ecology, and the opportunity it presented for seeing and working with patients in context.

The concept that an illness is experienced by the whole family was familiar. But our experience was based for the most part on work with families who came into therapy because they presented a psychological or psychosomatic member. We had little information about well functioning families under stress who were coping on their own. We were interested in the responses of families to the medical crisis, and the possibility of learning both from their spontaneous healing procedures and from the dysfunctional reactions that needed to be modified. The fact that patients came into the Cooperative Care unit with a care partner, usually a family member, provided a rare opportunity to study family strength and adaptation.

We interviewed 20 families, choosing middle-aged cancer patients who came into the unit with their spouses, and who had late adolescent or young adult children in the geographical area. We first saw the couple in the hospital, then met with the extended family and the couple for a second session outside the hospital, in our office, or their home. Using an open-ended format, we asked how they experienced the illness and its treatment, and what had changed in the family since the onset of this crisis. We tapped the ways in which they understood the illness, reorganized family patterns to cope, and made contact with medical and community resources.

In the following section, we report some of the characteristics of these viable families. We found both typical patterns and considerable variability. On one matter, however, reactions were essentially unanimous. Patients and care partners were clearly positive about the Cooperative Care Center, reflecting the sense of inclusion and support that is the basic purpose of such a unit. The setting allowed a semblance of normality in the extent to which the patient could control the experience of life in the hospital. Even against the background of boredom and pain that frequently accompanies the confinement, patient and care partner could control time and the access to their territory, continue many of the usual patterns of discussion, complaint and nurturance, and mobilize the resources of family and friends in accordance with their own needs. It is an important factor, of course, that the middle aged couples we interviewed were usually partners in long term marriages, so that the care partner arrangement was familiar as well as desirable.

THE REORGANIZATION OF FAMILY PATTERNS

Every chronic illness challenges the family's established patterns, and the organization of the family must change in order to cope with the new reality. In the face of invasive medical procedures, the boundaries of the family become more permeable, and the family must deal with the challenge to their sense of privacy. As an illness progresses, a family frequently exhausts its resources, needing to expand the healing network to include other relatives and community help—a process that comes naturally to some families and is difficult for others. Within the immediate family, roles and patterns of interaction must reflect variations in the energy of the sick person and the balance of stress and resilience in the caregiver(s).

There are a number of factors that determine how a family will change in the face of serious illness: the developmental stage of the family; whether the patient is an adult or child; how he or she fits into the family's practical and emotional patterns; and the nature and course of the illness. In any circumstance, the challenge is to strike a balance between continuity and change. Effective adaptation usually involves flexibility in the way the family functions—in its ability to include a variety of perspectives without paralyzing conflict, to judge when it must find new patterns, and to hold to the familiar when that is comforting and still adaptive.

In the group we studied, the patients were adults with complex functions before the onset of the illness. They were breadwinners, homemakers, the ones who paid bills or managed the social calendar—functions that represented the practical chores and the division of labor in the home. But they also had particular functions in the patterns of family interaction: the tower of strength, the mediator in family quarrels, the one who diffused tension with jokes and amiability, or the one who was dependable in practical or emotional crises. Therefore, the systemic changes—the assumption of new roles and functions—was expressed in each family in idiosyncratic ways. In talking with the couple, we heard and observed how they functioned and what was changing. When we met with the whole family, we saw a more complex picture of family patterns, with significant implications for the way the illness was handled and how the family would deal with aftercare.

Our sample included patients whose prognosis was good as well as those with terminal cancer, and the adaptation of the family inevitably varied as a function of this reality. However, all families dealt with the periodic discomfort of the chemotherapy treatments, and the need to fill in for a period, then recognize the moment when it was possible and advisable to cede functions again to the patient.

The core issue in any situation with a chronically or seriously ill family member is to balance protection and autonomy. Since the capacity of the patient fluctuated as a function of the illness and the medical procedures, family members needed to gauge the needs and understand when they changed—a task that is extremely difficult. All the families in the study were struggling with this issue, in their own terms. Patients and care partners, for instance, were concerned with the functions that had to be taken over: cooking, housecleaning, paying bills. They were aware of the pain experienced by the patient when long-term chores were relinquished, as well as the burden imposed on the caregiver. One woman commented that she had to learn how to use a checkbook and to find out where important papers were kept, and that she knew that was stressful for her husband. They described how they had talked about it together, and how his distress was balanced by his need to know that she would be able to manage alone, if necessary.

At the developmental stage of these families, we also found many adaptations in the relationship between the two adult generations, in the pattern of closeness and distance, and in the participation in decisionmaking. At a stage when the parents had been autonomously functioning and the offspring were building their independent lives and their own families, the boundaries between generations had been appropriately firm. With the onset of a parent's illness, concern for the patient and for the burden on the other parent brought the younger generation closer, in most cases. The grown children also tended to take a more active role than formerly in practical matters and in the discussion of medical options.

As we have noted elsewhere (Minuchin & Minuchin, 1987), the key to successful adaptation lies in calibration: the orchestration of moves to be helpful, the willingness to convey reactions openly, and the ability to modify behavior in keeping with feedback. One adult son was reluctant to invade his father's privacy in the shower, though he knew that the older man was dangerously frail. He was greatly relieved when his father asked his help, but needed to adapt again when he tried to button his father's shirt, after the shower, and his father waved him off. This simple episode embodied a workable cycle of signals, responses, and adaptations. In another case, the patient was embarrassed by the baldness that resulted from chemotherapy and was protective of the feelings of her children, always wearing a wig in their presence. When her son came into the room unexpectedly one day while she was bareheaded, she grabbed for the wig, but he said casually, "It's okay, Mom." She commented in the interview that she had laughed and relaxed, and that she had not been concerned since that day about whether the children saw her without the wig.

These are the micromovements of daily life. It requires an effort to change customary patterns, to be sensitive and protective without rendering the patient helpless, and to allow others to help when it is needed. It means picking up cues about what is needed and acceptable, and being alert to whether these conditions are different today than yesterday. It is a difficult task, even for the relatively viable families we interviewed, and it must be accomplished against a background of fear and stress. It is important for the hospital staff to notice how the family is managing, to gather information on what has been changing, and to register the complaints that signal failure in the efforts to calibrate change effectively. The Cooperative Care Unit is a particularly useful setting for maximizing contact between staff and family, and allowing for the recognition and support of constructive efforts to care for the patient and cope with change.

THE MEANING OF ILLNESS

Though all the families in our study would accept general scientific formulations about disease, the meaning of the illness was more personal and idiosyncratic. These families needed to make sense of what was happening, beyond the scientific facts, and their explanations came from their value systems and family history. Several families considered it the will of God, or some version of Fate, though the implications varied. One family was accepting in a relatively passive way, depending on prayer and faith. Another equally religious family balanced their belief that "God will take care of Harold" with very active efforts to meet new realities and mobilize family and friends, functioning in a kind of collaborative relationship with higher powers. For a family in which ovarian cancer had a three-generational history and was always fatal, the meaning of the illness was all too clear. In this case, the depressive sense of inevitability was offset in part by the patient's humor, her husband's energetic optimism, and the protective efforts of the parents to mediate the despair of the adolescent children. For this couple, also, the fact that the daughter was adopted was a comfort, given their understanding of the connection between heredity and disease.

Though there may be a shared family view about the illness, individual members do not all relate to the patient in the same way. In their study of families with handicapped children, Sigel, Stinson, and Flaugher (1993) noted that parents often had shared beliefs about the meaning and handling of the child's condition but differed nonetheless in the behavioral expression of those beliefs. Their findings highlight gender, both of parent and child, as a crucial determinant. This is, of course, an important factor in all families and situations. However, the information from our families suggests that the point is broader. The way in which different family members relate to the patient has much to do with long-term relationships, the previous role of the patient in the family, and the personality and style of each individual. Women may be statistically more protective in their behavior and men more down-to-earth, but we have seen many reversals of that pattern, within and across generations, as families manage, reorganize, and change in the face of crisis.

In all of the families studied, the sense of time took on a new experiential dimension. The present became the place where the family lived, and the effort was to slow time down. Since the future was uncertain, in very serious cases the tendency was often to focus on the past. Frequently there was a rosy tint to old memories, but sometimes old grievances came to the fore, with a strong need to resolve them while there was still time and to expiate guilt and ask forgiveness. That can be a positive process. A pervasive refusal to look at the future, however, has a toxic quality for the patient. The implicit message in this denial is the premature burial of the sick member, since the future is excluded. When we identified this type of transaction, we responded therapeutically by exploring incomplete tasks in family relationships and viable functions that could involve the patient, e.g. the sick father could teach math to the older daughter. The goal was to keep time flowing—to indicate the possibilities that still remained and the significance of future moments.

It has been suggested that an individual goes through particular stages in facing a terminal illness and death: that denial, anger and resistance precede acceptance. But the experience is undoubtedly more complex, involving the whole family and reflecting many factors that militate against an invariable sequence. The progress of the disease is relevant, and so is the organization of the family and the adaptation of its members as conditions change. Various studies have suggested, for instance, that some families tend to marginalize the patient as time passes, focusing increasingly on the normal issues of life and involving the patient less in activities and decisions. That form of adaptation contributes to negative prognoses and death (Cole & Reiss, 1993). Families may also have different cycles of vulnerability and strength. Some mobilize effectively at the onset of the crisis, but have difficulty sustaining themselves for the long haul, while others are shocked and disorganized by the crisis but are able to regroup for consistent long-term care. It is important for physicians and support staff to recognize the style of a particular family, and to monitor the potential for difficulties in their adaptations over time.

CONCLUSIONS

Through its request for a care partner, the Cooperative Care Center opens the door of the hospital to the family. Its implications go far beyond the immediate, helpful, and cost-effective functions of the partner in the hospital setting. Cooperative Care offers the possibility for implementing a true biopsychosocial model of medicine. In our view, it is the necessary structure for the practice of family medicine within a hospital setting.

What are the Advantages of This Model?

The advantages begin at the point of entry, in that the selection of the partner is in the hands of the patient. The definition of significant people is dictated not by society, but by the rules of intimacy. The choice is apt to be a family member, but the definition of family is broad, including very close friends or lovers. The important point is that the patient comes into the hospital with a person to whom he or she is connected, and that this person is a gateway to the larger, intimate network of people who are concerned with the patient and who will be involved in aftercare.

The setting and the manner in which the unit functions empowers this network. Care partners are not dismissed when the patient enters and summoned back at discharge. They are involved in the cycle of evaluation and treatment. They are informed, they have input, and they have functions. When the care partner leaves with the patient, caretaking at home can be confident and effective, both in medical and psychological terms.

In this setting, also, anamnesis becomes more than history-taking. It involves the perspectives and experiences of different people, and the observation of the place of the patient in his or her normal context. A sequence of two interviews is the most effective method for understanding the meaning of the disease and how it is being handled. In the first interview, with patient and care partner, it is possible to gather information, observe their relationship, and find out who they consider to be the other significant people in the larger family network. A second interview, including these significant people, expands understanding to an even more realistic level, clarifying the customary patterns of the family (however "family" is defined) and its current adaptations. Who has taken over functions for the patient? What is the style of the family in telling its story? Who provides backup for the care partner? How are decisions made? What expectations do different members have about the illness? Is there a family member besides the care partner who is an essential contact for the medical staff? Are there alliances, coalitions, or disagreements in the family? Are they manageable, or do they stress the patient and jeopardize compliance with the medical regimen when the patient is at home? The two-stage process yields a rich diagnosis: of family patterns as the context for the patient and the handling of the illness. In the Cooperative Care Unit, such a process can be easily implemented by the staff of the Education Center.

The procedures in the Education Center also permit an interactive way of discussing the nature of the illness and the details of care. Discussions with patient, partner, and relevant family members militate against the kind of protective secrecy that is instinctive in some families and that is actually a burden for the patient. The process of listening and raising questions in the family group also clarifies the roles of family members for aftercare, and increases their sense of responsibility and commitment to the patient. At the same time, the discussions build a healing partnership between family members and the medical team.

Finally, the knowledge gained in the Cooperative Care Unit about how a family functions allows for a differentiated home care program. It is possible to predict how the family will manage at home while patient and partner are still in the hospital, and with that knowledge, to construct a regime that recognizes the likely pattern of response and is shaped toward maximum compliance with medical necessities.

In general, the Cooperative Care setting and organizational structure represent a major step forward in combining effective medical care with the realities of the patient's social context. It is also the kind of setting in which the potential for ongoing collaboration between the medical team and family-oriented professionals can best be realized.

6

THE PROFESSIONAL STAFF'S PERSPECTIVE

Shirley A. Garnett, Kimberly S. Glassman, and Anthony J. Grieco

---

The professional staff of the Cooperative Care Unit includes the physicians who see the patients regularly and are responsible for their primary care; the Therapeutic Center's nurse-clinicians, who provide around-the-clock patient care and supervise the diagnostic and therapeutic regimen while the patient is hospitalized; and the Education Center's nurse-educators, nutritionists, social workers, and pharmacists. This multi disciplinary team is responsible for orientation to Cooperative Care on admission, insuring an adequate care partner, and providing and evaluating educational services for patients and care partners during hospitalization.

The AIDS Support Team consists of an AIDS Nurse Clinical Specialist and a Senior Social Worker. Together they are responsible for the most complex AIDS patients and for establishing and interpreting standards of practice for the staffs of both Cooperative Care and the traditional hospital.

The support staff in the Therapeutic Center includes a clerical staff, who greet patients and attend to their housekeeping and maintenance questions, arrange appointments and escort service to Radiology and Laboratories, and handle the chart document. Charting is done via computer in Cooperative Care. Support staff tasks therefore include insertion of hard copies from the computer printer, organization of the chart, and delivery to Medical Records after the patient is discharged. A supply aide maintains an adequate amount of medical/surgical supplies and stationery for the unit.

The support staff in the Education Center includes a secretary/receptionist who greets the patients, shows them the orientation film if appropriate, calls to remind them of appointments with the professional staff, maintains records of patient participation, and handles all phone calls coming into the Education Center. A clerk maintains supplies of materials and handles photocopying as well as duplication through the Printing Services Department.

An Administrative Secretary handles the Education Center payroll and employee recordkeeping as well as all phone calls, typing and other administrative responsibilities for the Administrative Staff.

A Logistics Manager is in charge of the nonmedical aspects of the Department. She monitors the budget, handles purchasing and repairs, and insures a safe and comfortable environment for the patients.

THE EDUCATION CENTER

The Education Center is where the process of developing a somewhat apprehensive patient and spouse or friend into a Cooperative Care patient and care partner begins.

After the admission process, the patient and care partner begin their orientation in the Education Center by viewing a videotape which describes the physical set up and philosophy of Cooperative Care. Following the video viewing, a nurse-educator sits down with them in a quiet carrel.

She introduces herself and begins to get acquainted and make them feel at ease. She completes an admission form by using the information they give her. While completing this "history," she also is formulating a plan for the patient's education: identifying appropriate classes with a nurse-educator, referrals that should be made for nutrition education, medication counseling with a pharmacist, and stress reduction and relaxation. These recommendations go onto the patient cardex and are completed and documented on the chart during hospitalization. A schedule of appointments is made for each patient and hung on their door during the night.

The Education Center is staffed 7 days a week from 8:30 A.M. to 5:30 P.M. Staffing usually is lighter on Saturday, but heavier on Sunday, to accommodate the usual high number of admissions that day.

All members of the Education Center professional staff are Master's-prepared and are of senior level. They are able to assess patients' needs and act to meet them independently. Each of the disciplines represented in the Education Center staff has a specific expertise. We will look at each discipline in turn and the role each plays in the education of the patient and care partner.

Nurse Educator

We have stated that orientation to Cooperative Care, putting the patient at ease, and formulating a plan of education are the nurse-educator's first responsibilities. Subsequently, she carries out the plan of education. Most educational sessions are carried out on a one-to-one, or more accurately a one-to-two, basis, including both patient and care partner.

Classes are offered frequently on cardiac risk reduction, care of the Hickman catheter, Type I and Type II Diabetes and all the associated education required, including self-injection technique, high and low blood sugar, how to prevent a hypoglycemic reaction and what to do in the event that one occurs, and proper skin and foot care. The nurse will refer the patient and care partner to the Education Center nutritionist and reinforce the importance of proper diet in good diabetes control.

Nutritionist

The nutritionist assesses the nutrition education needs of patients and counsels in all areas of diet and nutrition which will help the patient. She acts on referrals from physicians, nurse-educators in the Education Center and senior nurse clinicians in the Therapeutic Center. She also monitors the admission lists for patients seen before, and those who she suspects might benefit from diet counseling.

The role of diet in diabetes control is clearly accepted, but many patients need increased understanding and reinforcement in this area. When appropriate, the nutritionist also counsels on cardiac risk reduction diets, weight control, and appropriate diet during chemotherapy and radiation treatments. She advises AIDS patients on supporting their increased nutritional needs, particularly when mouth sores and/ or diarrhea impact negatively on nutritional status. Food preparation to avoid GI infections in the immunodepressed patient is discussed.

If the nutritionist and the patient think additional education is necessary after discharge, an appointment can be made with the outpatient nutritionist for follow-up.

Nutrition education is given a great deal of emphasis in Cooperative Care. This reflects not only the important role nutrition plays in recovery and disease prevention, but also the welter of misinformation which is available. It is an area in which patients freely ask for advice and help. Perhaps this reflects the patient's understanding that only he controls what he eats and that this has a bearing on his regaining and maintaining a healthy status.

Social Worker

There are situations over which patients can have no control, such as in a terminal or prolonged illness. In these situations, the skills of the social worker may be called upon to help with emotional adjustment. Social workers will see all patients when suicide is a possibility or when abuse is suspected. They work closely with the care partner and other family members, aware that serious illness impacts severely on the whole family, and that the support and understanding of all those involved is very important to the wellbeing of the patient.

Like the nutritionist, the social worker acts on referrals from the physician, the senior nurse-clinician and the nurse-educator. She, too, checks the admission list for patients known to her from prior admissions.

Pharmacist

A pharmacist sits down with each patient and care partner who have been identified as able to benefit from help with their medications. This is done to insure that the patient knows the action of each medication and understands how and when the medications should be taken, what to do in case of a missed dose, and any side effects that should be reported to the physician. During the consultation the pharmacist explores all the medications the patient is taking, and is alert for possible drug interactions.

THE THERAPEUTIC CENTER

At the time of their appointment, the patient and care partner come from their own hospital room, locking the door behind them, to a centralized area where they are seen by their nurse in an examination room. She does a physical assessment, administers treatments, checks on the patient's medical progress, and identifies additional educational and psychological needs. She reports to the physician by phone or through chart documentation. Physicians regularly visit their patients and depend on the nurses for observation between times, as there are no house staff in Cooperative Care except in an emergency, when they are always available.

If educational and psychosocial needs are observed, the senior nurse-clinician refers the patient to the Education Center, where the staff of nurse-educators, nutritionists, social workers, and pharmacists meet with the patient and care partner to assist them in their particular area of expertise.

After consultation with a pharmacist or nurse to insure understanding, the patient is put on Self-Administration of Medications (SAM). The nurse dispenses a supply of medication sufficient for a day or two. The patient takes his own medications; the care partner provides assistance if necessary. This is reported to his nurse, who documents on the chart what medications were taken and when, as reported by the patient.

Therapeutic Center Staffing

The staff in the Therapeutic Center are Senior Nurse-Clinicians. This means they have reached the top rung of the clinical ladder. They are experienced and competent clinicians, who are able to assess their patient's condition accurately and make good clinical judgements.

Most of the nurses have Master's Degrees and many years of experience. Many have backgrounds in critical care nursing, as has the Director of Nursing of Cooperative Care.

They are responsible for around-the-clock care and meet with their patients on an appointment basis. The patient and care partner come to the Therapeutic Center for their examinations as frequently as they think necessary, with twice a day as a minimum. The nurse checks the medication record which the patient has kept, dispensing additional medications as needed.

CONCLUSION

The multidisciplinary team of professionals, comprising the attending physicians, nurse clinicians, nurse-educators, nutritionists, social workers, pharmacists, and others, provide comprehensive services to patients in Cooperative Care in a delivery system which is based upon the active participation of effective care partners. The unit would not work so well if any cog were omitted.

In the next section of this book, each chapter will provide further details about the professional staff, their viewpoints, how they select patients, and how they provide medical care, nursing care and education, as well as their techniques for assuring patient safety.

7

PATIENT SELECTION

Jeanne Dzurenko, Kimberly S. Glassman, and
Anthony J. Grieco

SOURCES OF PATIENT ENTRY

Proper selection of patients is essential for the success of a Cooperative Care Unit. The central prerequisite for admission to Cooperative
Care is the necessity for acute care hospitalization, namely, that the
medical treatment cannot be provided safely at home, although it
might not require continuous 24-hour bedside nursing or intensive
care level monitoring.

Admissions to Cooperative Care come from three sources: scheduled
direct admissions, transfers from other inpatient units of the hospital,
and urgent admissions from the Emergency Room. The attending physician makes the initial determination that the medical regimen can
safely be administered within the Cooperative Care setting. To assist
physicians in making that determination, the Cooperative Care medical director and nursing leadership are available to give advice when
there are specific debatable circumstances.

A detailed list of specific admission criteria is not used; rather simple guidelines are provided: the patient must be sick enough to require
acute care hospitalization, the patient must be mobile enough for the

care partner to be able to handle personal needs in the room and transfers to the centralized services, the medical condition must be stable enough so that intensive care unit monitoring is not required, and an adequate care partner must be available.

Of course, the patient and family must feel comfortable within the environment, as this ultimately determines whether treatment in Cooperative Care will become an acceptable option.

Routine admissions are scheduled via the Admitting Office. These patients and their families know in advance that their care will be provided in the Cooperative Care environment. At the time arrangements for admission are made, the physician or the office staff inform the patient of the need for a care partner. Included among the mix of routine admissions are oncology patients, people requiring invasive diagnostic procedures such as cardiac catheterization, and patients who require medical care with nursing supervision; for example, people with extremely poorly controlled insulin-dependent diabetes. Frequently encountered diagnostic groups include patients with acquired immunodeficiency syndrome, and those with cardiopulmonary diseases or neurological disorders.

Transfers from other inpatient hospital units of Tisch Hospital comprise barely 5% of the bed-base in Cooperative Care. This group includes surgical patients who are in the early postoperative stage, particularly those with medical or surgical complications requiring longer observation and treatment than usual. During the postoperative Cooperative Care stay, not only will the patients undergo the usual treatments and medication titration, but also comprehensive instruction about their care, as is true of other categories of patients in the unit. During this period of the postoperative hospitalization there will be further medication adjustments and education about wound care or instruction about a new aspect of daily care, with the expectation that the patient and care partner will take an active role in these treatments early during the hospitalization.

For example, postoperative coronary artery bypass grafting patients typically will be transferred to Cooperative Care during the last few days of their hospitalization. Here, the nursing staff teach wound care, and they continue to reinforce the appropriate medication schedule and monitor the progression of independence and participation in care.

The Cooperative Care environment empowers the "significant other" to experience the postoperative phase in a home like environment, with the comfort of knowing that the professional staff is in the wings, but not at the bedside. Reducing the anxiety of going home after a worrisome hospitalization is a prime goal of Cooperative Care.

Many patients who are admitted to the hospital begin their treatment in an Emergency Room. These patients may enter the Emergency Room with the chief complaint of high fever, chest pain, or shortness of breath. After triage, the initial diagnostic evaluation is completed by the attending physician and the Emergency Room physicians. If inpatient admission is required, the Emergency Room nursing leadership and medical staff will assess the patient and, when appropriate, suggest Cooperative Care as an option to the attending physician.

ONCOLOGY PATIENTS

Oncology patients make up approximately 25% of the Cooperative Care population. These patients require cyclical chemotherapy administration which cannot routinely be given in the physician's office. The Cooperative Care setting provides not only hospital services, but the added support of the family member or friend who stays with the patient as the care partner. In addition, the patient is assigned to an Oncology Nurse Specialist (ONS) during the initial oncology hospitalization. The ONS will participate in the treatment of the patient every month for the duration of the illness. The ONS, in caring for the patient, administers the chemotherapy, monitors blood values, and helps to determine the plan of care in collaboration with the attending physician. Intravenous drips and boluses are administered according to specific protocols. Later in the day and night, antiemetics are administered by the nurse-clinician as needed. Continuity of care is maintained over the months of treatment, since each patient who returns to Cooperative Care for therapy is followed by the same ONS.

If the oncology patient were admitted to the conventional part of the hospital for treatment, he or she might enter a different nursing unit each month. That might mean a different nursing staff and a different medical house staff each month. In Cooperative Care, by maintaining continuity of the treating team, including the ONS, the patient's anxiety level is reduced, thereby optimizing patient satisfaction.

Of course, chemotherapeutic regimens vary from patient to patient and from diagnosis to diagnosis. Lymphoma, lung cancer, colon cancer, ovarian cancer and pancreatic cancer are some of the more common malignancies treated in the Cooperative Care setting. Duration of the chemotherapy infusion cycle varies from as little as 1 to 3 days to as long as a 7-day continuous intravenous infusion.

INVASIVE PROCEDURES

Patients requiring invasive diagnostic procedures as part of their workups are another group which Cooperative Care serves. These people usually require a 1- or 2-day stay. Procedure patients handled by Cooperative Care include those undergoing cardiac catheterization, bronchoscopy, myelograms and liver biopsies, among other procedures. In most instances, these patients undergo preadmission testing and education at the Cooperative Care Education Center within one week of the scheduled admission. They then enter the unit on the morning of the procedure. The Cooperative Care staff evaluates them, sends them to the procedure, and afterwards provides recovery-room like care in the observation room.

The Cooperative Care observation room has six beds, staffed by two registered nurses. This setup allows for close monitoring, which is scheduled for up to 6 hours postprocedure, depending upon the predicted need. During the recovery period of observation, bed rest is maintained, strict intake and output is measured, and frequent monitoring of vital signs is provided. Care partners are incorporated into the observation room pattern of care, and remain at the bedside during most of the postprocedure period. As auxiliary members of the caring team in the observation unit, care partners are engaged in watching the patient, assisting with meals, and providing emotional support. Postprocedure care guidelines are reinforced with both the patient and care partner so that both will feel comfortable later when they are in their room without direct professional nursing supervision. Approximately 4 hours after the patient leaves the observation room, a nurse-clinician will perform a physical assessment in the patient's room.

PATIENTS WITH AIDS

The acquired immunodeficiency syndrome (AIDS) epidemic has had a profound impact upon health care services world wide. Patients afflicted with AIDS have complex medical, nursing, and psychosocial needs. The Cooperative Care environment can provide all aspects of care for these people, while maintaining their dignity and fostering independence. From the onset of the disease, to the first opportunistic infections, to the end stage of the disease, Cooperative Care allows patients to learn in great detail about their disease, the drugs used to treat its manifestations, and techniques of self-care. Care partners are motivated to participate in those teaching sessions.

Patients with AIDS account for approximately 25% of the 104–bed Cooperative Care census. With their complex clinical needs and extensive educational needs, this population fits in well in Cooperative Care. Although they are quite ill, by and large these patients are strongly motivated to be as independent as possible in their care. They are usually very eager to become thoroughly educated about their disease process and their treatment. In addition, AIDS patients generally have quite strong support systems of family and friends, and manage well in this patient-centered environment.

The infectious disease specialists managing AIDS patients select those with a high severity of illness for admission to Cooperative Care. With the assistance of the care partner, this very ill population has been extremely successfully handled in Cooperative Care's patient-centered environment. By learning to participate in care early in the hospitalization, AIDS patients become more acclimated to the complex lifestyle changes that result from the disease. Anemia, leukopenia, intercurrent *Pneumocystis carinii* pneumonia (PCP), and malnutrition require careful management by professionals, but the patient's involvement in awareness helps. Recently, a Cooperative Care patient who was hospitalized for a different manifestation of AIDS announced, "I have PCP and need to start pentamidine immediately." He was, indeed, the first to make the diagnosis of PCP in himself, as soon as he developed cough and shortness of breath. His dramatic statement expedited his care, and treatment started within minutes of his announcement.

During the years of this epidemic, the education center has developed a specific AIDS-related curriculum. This helps to accomplish the goal of having the patient, care partner, friends, and family understand and face the challenges that are present or on the horizon. Technical instruction is part of this package. For example, care of a Hickman catheter and handling total parenteral nutrition (TPN) administration are two classes frequently attended by AIDS patients. During a Cooperative Care stay, patients may need to learn how to administer subcutaneous injections of erythropoietin and colony-stimulating factors, intravenous infusions for home aftercare, and other technical tasks as well.

Through collaboration between nutritionists, pharmacists, and physicians who treat AIDS patients requiring TPN, Cooperative Care has become a nearly perfect setting for the delivery of TPN. Before the first patient receiving TPN was admitted to Cooperative Care, a policy and procedure was outlined describing the educational classes, the methods for ordering TPN in the hospital computer system, and the procedure for the initial administration of TPN. Care partners for these patients were considered to be of paramount importance, both during the class and during the administration itself. An initial bag of TPN solution is infused overnight, with the patient housed in the observation room and the care partner present. This allows the nurse to evaluate the patient's tolerance for TPN, and gives the care partner an opportunity to observe the process in operation. If the patient tolerates the infusion, it is expected that all following bags of TPN will be administered each night in the patient's room, with only the patient and care partner in attendance.

OTHER MEDICAL DIAGNOSES

Patients with other medical diagnoses, such as insulin-requiring diabetes, congestive heart failure, or pneumonia, also can be managed effectively within the Cooperative Care setting. In all cases, the focus must remain on the ability of the patient and care partner to function within this environment. The patient should be willing to take part in his or her care. In addition, the care partner must be an active participant in the patient's plan of care.

The traditional hospital setting inhibits patient control and decisionmaking. Cooperative Care focuses on the patient's needs, and encourages an interactive relationship between the professional staff and the patient.

Cardiac Catheterization

Cardiac catheterizations are most frequently performed as outpatient procedures. However, some patients require admission, with the procedure performed the day of entry, and others undergo catheterization as part of a hospitalization for treatment of the underlying cardiac disorder.

Whether the patient is scheduled for outpatient or inpatient catheterization is obviously the determination of the attending physician. The outpatients have prescheduled observation room time following their procedures, and undergo preadmission testing. On the day of the preadmission testing, the patients attend a class in the Education Center regarding pre-and postprocedure care. Patients arrive at the cardiac catheterization lab on the morning of the procedure and, although they are not yet on the unit, they are assigned a bed in Cooperative Care. Following the procedure, the patient is returned to the observation room in Cooperative Care and recovers for approximately 4 hours, during which frequent vital signs are followed and intake and output are measured. Once the patient has recovered, he or she spends another 4 to 6 hours in a patient room until the physician clears them for discharge home. If complications arise, the room is available for admission if necessary.

Same-day cardiac catheterizations differ from outpatient cardiac catheterizations in several ways. These patients are admitted directly to Cooperative Care the day of the procedure. However, in anticipation of entry, they have already been to preadmission testing and to the education center for preadmission education, following the same protocol as does the outpatient. Upon arrival on the day of the catheterization, they are assigned a patient room, are evaluated, then instructed to wait in the room until they are called for the procedure. Postprocedure recovery is the same as for outpatients, except that the patient will remain overnight in Cooperative Care. If stable, the physician will discharge the patient in the morning, unless urgent surgery or other compelling treatment is indicated.

Finally, patients undergoing cardiac catheterization during the course of hospitalization for treatment of complications of the underlying disease, such as congestive heart failure or unstable angina, are scheduled for postprocedure observation room time in the same way.

If complications arise, such as the need for continuous monitoring, necessitating transfer to the Intensive Care Unit, arrangements are made for the patient to go there overnight. Once the patient stabilizes, he or she may be returned to Cooperative Care directly from the Intensive Care Unit.

Liver Biopsy

In most instances, liver biopsies do not require an overnight hospital stay. Cooperative Care handles these patients as outpatients. As in the case of cardiac catheterizations, patients scheduled for liver biopsies attend preprocedure educational sessions and preprocedure testing within 7 days of the biopsy. Patients arrive on the unit the morning of the procedure, are evaluated, then assigned a room. They proceed directly to the observation unit, where the biopsy is performed. Once the procedure is completed, the patient spends approximately 4 hours in the observation room on strict bedrest, with vital signs being monitored closely during those 4 hours. Two hemograms are drawn during the first 4 hours postprocedure. The patient is then released from the observation room, but continues strict bedrest in the patient room with his or her care partner. If the patient remains stable and the hematocrit remains satisfactory, the patient is discharged home that evening.

Lupus Nephritis

Patients with systemic lupus erythematosus complicated by active ne-
phritis often require pulse therapy of intravenous cyclophosphamide.
During the brief Cooperative Care hospitalization to accomplish this,
they receive 1 or 2 liters of intravenous fluid in addition to the cyclophosphamide. Handling potential fluid or electrolyte imbalances,
nausea or vomiting, monitoring vital signs, treating side effects, measuring intake and output, is accomplished in the observation room
overnight.

CONCLUSION

Patients selected for admission to Cooperative Care are no different
from those who are to be admitted to traditional hospital units. Proper
selection of patients requires that the physician be attentive to the
likelihood that, for periods of time, the patient will be safely observed
by a motivated family member or friend acting as a care partner. The
details of the medical illness are less important in the selection process than is the level of nursing care needed and the latitude possible
for providing that care. If constant bedside nursing is required for periods of time which can be absorbed into the observation room schedule,
then the intensity of illness can be safely handled. In the case of an
acutely ill patient, supported by a care partner who is able to perform
the inroom daily living functions and transfers, and mobile enough
with that assistance to have the professionals' ministrations occur in
the centralized core services area, Cooperative Care is often the best
site for inpatient care delivery.

8

MEDICAL: THE PATIENT WITH CARDIOVASCULAR DISEASE

Sydney J. Mehl

Cooperative Care offers unique opportunities for the evaluation and management of patients with cardiovascular disease. Usually, cardiac symptoms are related to activity; therefore, therapies that are deemed to be effective in the traditional hospital setting, with the patient mostly at rest or with some limited ambulation in the hospital corridors, may fall far short of expected goals when the patient becomes more ambulatory and independent. Cooperative Care allows better titration of various cardiovascular therapies since it enables us to observe patients in a more ambulatory atmosphere, where they and their care partners are more active participants in therapy and assume more independent functions. Quality of Life issues, which are assuming an increasingly important focus in today's medical environment, are thus more apt to be addressed than in the traditional hospital setting.

Many cardiac patients go through a series of stages, ranging from very critical to relatively stable. Thus, the patient with ischemic heart disease may enter the hospital with an acute myocardial infarction or unstable angina, and progress through stages in which he or she becomes increasingly more stable and less dependent on high levels of monitoring and nursing care. In parallel with this, the patient may require treatment in a critical care unit, then move on to a step-down unit, a traditional hospital nursing unit, Cooperative Care, and further outpatient evaluation and management. Of course, not every patient will need to pass through all of these hospital areas, or in the same sequence.

Patients with a variety of cardiovascular diseases and problems are excellent candidates for Cooperative Care, with some clear-cut exceptions. The operative words are *patient selection, modification* and *flexibility* in care.

Many cardiac patients have a variety of interrelated problems and diagnoses, but it may be helpful to look at individual diagnostic related groupings in the Cooperative Care setting.

THE PATIENT WITH ISCHEMIC HEART DISEASE

Ischemic heart disease is certainly the most common of cardiac diagnoses, and can involve evaluation and management issues related to acute myocardial infarction and various degrees of angina pectoris. The approach to patients with atherosclerotic heart disease has evolved rapidly in the past decade, and includes medical therapies, catheter-interventional therapies, surgical revascularization, and life style changes. A patient who is known or suspected of having an acute myocardial infarction is clearly not a candidate for Cooperative Care. Such patients are best treated in a critical care unit with consideration given to pharmacological or mechanical reperfusion, limitation of infarct size, treatment of life-threatening arrhythmias, shock, etc. After a period of stability, the patient may be transferred to a step-down unit or to a traditional hospital nursing area for continued care. Transfer to Cooperative Care can be considered at any point, depending on the level of monitoring needed. In Cooperative Care almost all standard post-MI therapies may be modified and implemented. Other patients with ischemic heart disease may come to Cooperative Care via other routes:

Coronary angiography in the past has traditionally been an inpatient procedure, but with current utilization/practice management guidelines, most patients requiring elective studies are treated as out-patients. On occasion, a patient admitted for an outpatient study may have to be admitted to Cooperative Care due to postcatheterization problems such as excessive bleeding from puncture sites, contrast dye reactions, or prolonged procedures that go on until late in the day.

Also, based on the results of coronary angiography, some patients may need to stay in the hospital for further interventional, medical, or surgical therapies. Patients with concurrent medical problems, such as anticoagulant therapy, diabetes, renal disease, or cerebrovascular dis-ease may need to be admitted before their procedure, and Cooperative Care often is utilized. In patients having an elective percutaneous transluminal coronary angioplasty or coronary atherectomy, a stay overnight in Cooperative Care usually is necessary after the procedure.

Patients who are admitted to the emergency room with chest pain who are "ruled out for having an acute myocardial infarction" are of-ten admitted to Cooperative Care for further evaluation and treat-ment. This may include titration of medical therapy, stress testing, and coronary angiography, as well as tests to determine if their pain was secondary to a non cardiac problem.

Patients may be transferred from the traditional hospital medical service for further titration of medical therapy and for progressive am-bulation prior to discharge home.

Patients may be transferred from the cardiovascular surgical service after coronary artery bypass surgery. Such patients often need titra-tion of medical therapy; wound care, usually to venotomy sites where veins were harvested for bypasses; sometimes parenteral antibiotics for wound infections, and progressive ambulation. Educational/life-style changes may be implemented in Cooperative Care as well.

Among the medical therapies employed in the treatment of the pa-tient with ischemic heart disease are anticoagulants, betablockers, calcium channel entry blockers, nitrates, angiotensin converting en-zyme (ACE) inhibitors, antiarrhythmic drugs, and lipid-lowering drugs. The Cooperative Care setting allows for unique titration and monitoring of these therapies, along with patient education.

Anticoagulation

Some patients recovering from an acute infarction may be candidates for anticoagulant therapy for several months or longer. These patients include those with certain atrial arrhythmias—in particular, atrial fi-brillation—and patients who are shown to have a left ventricular thrombus, usually on an echocardiographic study. Also, many clinicians prescribe anticoagulant therapy for several months in patients with large anterior infarctions. Heparin therapy can be accomplished by continuous infusion with the aid of a portable IV pump, which can be worn by the patient and programmed to deliver a dosage of heparin based on periodic determinations of the activated partial thromboplastin time (PTT). Coumadin usually is started concomitantly, and the dosage adjusted by following the prothrombin time (PT). Current recommendations suggest a therapeutic goal of between 1.3–1.5 X the control PT, to ensure adequate levels of anticoagulation while avoiding bleeding complications. Increasingly, the INR method of following the level of anticoagulation is being utilized. Education in the use of Coumadin is an extremely important objective that can be accomplished in Cooperative Care, as can arranging for follow up as an outpatient.

Beta Blockers

Numerous studies have demonstrated improved survival in patients given beta blockers after myocardial infarction. These drugs have long been a mainstay treatment for patients with angina pectoris. Dosage titration may be accomplished by careful monitoring of the heart rate and blood pressure, both at rest, and after activities of daily living. Also, patients and their care partners may be taught how to measure pulse and blood pressure, and parameters may be established for withholding doses based on unacceptably low readings.

Calcium Channel Entry Blockers

These are often used in patients with angina pectoris, and careful attention must be given to their effects on blood pressure and the heart rate.

Nitrates

These are also often used, in topical, oral, or sublingual forms. The main thing to watch with these drugs is their effect on blood pressure.

Angiotensin Converting Enzyme (ACE) Inhibitors

Studies suggesting improved survival in subsets of post-myocardial infarction patients treated with angiotensin converting enzyme inhibitors are in progress, and patients with ischemic heart disease and left ventricular systolic dysfunction have already been shown to benefit from angiotensin converting enzyme inhibitors. These drugs may cause unacceptable lowering of blood pressure, worsening renal function, and hyperkalemia. Thus, frequent blood pressure determinations are useful at the initiation of therapy, or when the dosage is raised, along with periodic monitoring of the BUN, creatinine, and electrolytes—all of which can be done easily and effectively in Cooperative Care.

Antiarrhythmic Medication

The results of the CAST study (Echt, Liebson, Mitchell et al., 1991) suggest that routine use of class I antiarrhythmic drugs in patients surviving myocardial infarction may be associated with *excess* mortality. Nevertheless, some patients with ischemic heart disease do require these drugs, and titration may be accomplished by frequent assessment of vital signs, ECG strips, Holter monitoring, and drug levels. Pro-arrhythmic effects usually (but not always) occur during the early stages of therapy, and may be heralded by more frequent extrasystoles noted by the nurse clinician on taking the vital signs; by worsening grades of arrhythmia detected by daily ECG recordings; or by periodic Holter monitoring. Some patients may require electrophysiological studies (EPS).

Lipid Lowering

During the stay at Cooperative Care, assessment of the patient's lipid profile may be done, and educational programs on the importance of diet in preventing the progression, and perhaps in helping regression of coronary atherosclerosis should be implemented. Some patients will, of course, need treatment with drugs to effect optimization of their lipid levels, and these can be started as well.

In summary, many patients with ischemic heart disease may be successfully managed, at various stages of their illness, in Cooperative Care, with benefits that may extend beyond those available with hospitalization in the traditional setting.

THE PATIENT WITH CONGESTIVE HEART FAILURE

Congestive heart failure (CHF) is one of the most common diagnostic related groupings for hospitalization, and Cooperative Care may be an optimal unit for managing many of these patients.

The patient presenting with acute pulmonary edema or CHF with significant hemodynamic instability is obviously not a candidate for direct admission to Cooperative Care, and usually requires stabilization in a critical care unit. Once they are stabilized, transfer to Cooperative Care is often possible and desirable. Most patients requiring hospitalization for management of CHF may be directly admitted to Cooperative Care. Typical treatment strategies involve the titration of various oral drug regimens, the use of intravenous diuretics when needed, and occasionally a "dobutamine holiday." The importance of salt restriction cannot be overemphasized, and a supervised sodium-restricted diet can be implemented in Cooperative Care, as can educational programs aimed at ensuring adequate sodium restriction when the patient is discharged.

Diuretics

Diuretics remain the most frequently used class of drugs for treating the fluid overload that is present in most patients with coronary heart failure. Increasing doses of oral diuretics demand careful monitoring of vital signs, along with daily weights, and sometimes assessment of inputs and outputs. In addition, careful follow up of renal function and electrolytes is necessary, especially monitoring of the serum potassium level. All of these modalities, along with periodic assessment of pulmonary rales and peripheral edema, are well accomplished in Cooperative Care. Often, the patient may become refractory to even large doses of oral diuretics such as furosemide and ethacrynic acid. In such cases, the use of metazolone, usually in combination with a loop diuretic, may result in significant diuresis. An all too frequent accompaniment is the development of severe hypokalemia. This can be treated with oral or parenteral potassium supplements, or addition of a potassium sparing diuretic such as spironolactone. Some clinicians advocate the use of continuous intravenous infusions of furosemide, which may be done in Cooperative Care using a portable programmable infusion pump.

Digitalis Preparations

Digitalis preparations are effective inotropic agents and may help the patient with congestive heart failure, particularly when the patient has a dilated left ventricle with diminished systolic function. Various schemes of oral or intravenous digitalization may be accomplished in Cooperative Care, along with periodic measurement of the serum drug level, and assessment of the ECG to look for toxicity.

Angiotensin Converting Enzyme (ACE) Inhibitors and Vasodilators

The concept of heart failure as a cardiocirculatory disorder has focused attention on the role of the peripheral circulatory vasoconstriction in, and perhaps "overcompensating" for, a diminished cardiac output, and contributing greatly to the deranged pathophysiology present. Thus, the use of agents that dilate the arterial and venous bed has been shown to alleviate symptoms of low output, and indeed prolong the survival of patients with heart failure. The initiation and titration of these drugs, including hydralazine, prazosin, nitrates, ACE inhibitors, and flosequinon, requires careful monitoring of the clinical response, and especially of their effect on systolic blood pressure. Oftentimes, the blood pressure will fall to levels thought to be dangerous. However, if evidence of improved cardiac output and subjective analysis of patient tolerance is present, this need not be a reason to withhold this important line of therapy. Certainly, hypotension that is symptomatic may contradict the aggressive use of these agents. With the ACE inhibitors, profound drops of blood pressure are sometimes noted, particularly in the patient who is overdiuresed. In addition, these drugs may have a worsening effect on renal function and may lead to problems with hyperkalemia. Thus, careful assessment of vital signs, and measurement of BUN, creatinine, and serum electrolytes is needed. Serial followups may lead to use of higher doses of these agents than would ordinarily be used when these drugs are begun on outpatients. Again, this is readily accomplished in Cooperative Care.

Beta-Blockers

Beta blockers were once almost always contraindicated in patients with heart failure, the exceptions being those patients who had predominantly diastolic dysfunction, those with obstructive cardiomyopathy, and those who needed control of the ventricular response in atrial fibrillation, when digitalis agents were ineffective alone. There is an emerging literature suggesting that chronic beta-blockade may improve symptoms, and perhaps survival, in certain subgroups of patients with diminished left ventricular systolic function and inappropriate activation of the neurohumoral system, leading to excessive levels of circulatory catecholamines, and perhaps an overcompensating tachycardia. The use of beta blockers in patients with heart failure obviously requires careful monitoring for worsening CHF, and Cooperative Care may be an ideal environment to judge the effects of this class of drugs both at rest and with increasing efforts that approach activities of daily life expected when patients are discharged.

Dobutamine Infusions

Some patients with heart failure benefit from a "dobutamine holiday" whereby infusion of the inotropic drug dobutamine for several days helps up-regulate beta receptors, and thus allow for improvement of heart failure when the infusion is terminated. Traditionally, patients who received these infusions had to be admitted to a critical care unit for careful monitoring, but now some selected patients are thought to be candidates for periodic infusion of dobutamine at home. Cooperative Care may be viewed as bridging the gap between infusion in an ICU and infusion in the patient's bedroom. The titration of the optimal dosage, and the response, both in terms of benefit and side effects, may be efficiently assessed in the Cooperative Care setting. The patient may then be able to get periodic infusions at home, or be readmitted to Cooperative Care at times when infusions are again necessary. The use of the portable, programmable infusion pump may make this therapy quite appropriate for Cooperative Care.

In those institutions where cardiac transplantation is done, Cooperative Care may be uniquely utilized in the extensive preoperative assessment, which includes detailed medical, social, and psychological evaluation. After the transplant, the patient may very much benefit from a stay in Cooperative Care where the numerous medications that must be taken, including powerful immunosuppressives, can be monitored, and their use explained to the patient. Education, both pre- and posttransplantation, is extremely important.

THE PATIENT WITH CARDIAC ARRHYTHMIAS

Cardiac arrhythmias are a common problem leading to hospital admissions, and Cooperative Care may be appropriate for those patients not requiring continuous on line monitoring. For patients who have ongoing, life-threatening or hemodynamically compromising arrhythmias, appropriate treatment is always given in critical care units.

Atrial Fibrillation

This is one of the most common arrhythmias, occurring in up to 10% of patients over the age of 70. It is associated with almost all forms of heart disease, but may also be a manifestation of a noncardiac disorder, such as hyperthyroidism. Occasionally, it occurs in the absence of demonstrable heart disease—lone atrial fibrillation. Hospitalization is often required to control a rapid ventricular response, particularly when the arrhythmia is first manifest, to begin parenteral anticoagulation—since atrial fibrillation is a leading cause of cerebral and systemic embolization—and to attempt conversion to sinus rhythm in selected patients.

Control of the ventricular response in patients who are otherwise not unstable is often an indication for Cooperative Care admission. Digitalis preparations, beta blockers, and calcium channel entry blockers may be used, either singularly or in combination. Periodic assessment of the apical rate can be accomplished by the nurse-clinician, by serial ECG recordings, and by serial Holter monitoring.

Anticoagulation is usually begun with intravenous heparin, and can be accomplished with the aid of portable, programmable infusion pumps, and monitoring of the partial thromboplastin time test (PTT). Warfarin therapy is often begun concomitantly, by mouth, and titrated until the prothrombin time (PT) or INR is in the therapeutic range. Education in the use of warfarin, and follow up monitoring strategies, are integral parts of anticoagulation that are done very well in Cooperative Care.

In selected patients, cardioversion, either with antiarrhythmic medication or electricity, is deemed desirable. Oftentimes, the patient is first begun on a regimen effective for rate control, anticoagulated, discharged, and readmitted several weeks later for electrical cardioversion. This is done to minimize the risk of thromboembolic complications. The procedure itself is often done in the electrophysiology laboratory, the cardiac catheterization laboratory, or the coronary care unit. Afterwards, the patient may be returned to Cooperative Care for further observation until discharge.

In rare cases when cardioversion is either not an option or unsuccessful, and antiarrhythmic drugs cannot adequately control a rapid ventricular response, radiofrequency AV nodal ablation may be done in the electrophysiology laboratory, followed by implantation of a permanent pacemaker. Afterwards, these patients may again be managed at Cooperative Care.

Sick Sinus Syndrome

This is the most common reason for pacemaker implantation in the United States. Criteria used to justify pacemaker implantation include significant bradycardia associated with symptoms such as syncope, lightheadedness, or extreme fatigue. A period of observation in Cooperative Care may be necessary to establish that these protean symptoms are indeed the result of bradycardia, and frequent assessment of the heart rate and rhythm and the correlation of rhythm slowing with the patients symptoms are well accomplished in Cooperative Care. Some patients suffer from the tachy-brady syndrome, in which the patient alternatively has rapid, usually supraventricular arrhythmias, and brady-arrhythmias. Drugs that effectively control the tachyarrhythmias may have a deleterious effect on the brady-arrhythmias, and antiarrhythmic drug therapy, together with permanent pacing, is often the solution. Usually the patient is transferred to the surgical service for pacemaker implantation, but then may benefit from aggressive management of periodic tachyarrhythmias back in Cooperative Care. Appropriate education regarding pacemaker follow up is well accomplished in Cooperative Care, and trans-telephonic pacemaker monitoring, which is usually the most effective means of pacemaker follow up, may be learned by patients and their health care partners.

Atrioventricular Block

This is another reason for pacemaker implantation, and selected patients may benefit from Cooperative Care for treatment of ancillary conditions, after pacemaker implantation.

Supraventricular Tachycardias

While relatively common, these do not usually require hospital admission for evaluation and treatment. In the patient with very frequent episodes, pharmacological antiarrhythmic therapy may be initiated in Cooperative Care. Also, in patients in whom an accessory AV pathway is present, which helps perpetuate frequent bouts of supraventricular tachycardia, radiofrequency ablation of the pathway may be performed, and the patient observed in Cooperative Care afterwards.

Ventricular Tachycardia and Ventricular Fibrillation

These arrhythmias are responsible for most cases of sudden cardiac death. In those patients who survive an out-of-hospital cardiac arrest, the 1-year mortality is unacceptably high. Strategies for therapeutic interventions include antiarrhythmic drug therapy based on the results of electrophysiological studies (EPS); rarely, catheter ablation techniques, and the use of the implantable cardioverter-defibrillator. Obviously, those patients just admitted after their cardiac arrest need monitoring and therapeutic interventions in a critical care unit. Other patients with serious ventricular arrhythmias may require evaluation of their arrhythmia and appropriate drug therapy based either on the results of serial Holter monitoring or EPS, and may be candidates for Cooperative Care. Examples are patients with high-grade ventricular ectopic activity, who are thought to be at significant risk for sudden cardiac death. The majority of these patients include those with ischemic heart disease, diminished left ventricular systolic function, and non sustained ventricular tachycardia.

THE PATIENT WITH UNEXPLAINED SYNCOPE

The evaluation of the patient with syncope of undetermined etiology usually involves evaluation of the cardiovascular and neurological systems. Workups that can be done in Cooperative Care include Holter monitoring, echocardiography (including trans esophageal echocardiography), tilt-table testing (to look for vasodepressor syncope), the determination of supine and upright blood pressure readings (to evaluate the role of postural hypotension), electroencephalography, and various modalities for imaging the brain (CT, MRI).

THE PATIENT WITH HYPERTENSION

Most hypertensive patients are diagnosed and treated in the ambulatory care setting. Those presenting with hypertensive crises in which acute effects of severely elevated blood pressure are manifest in the central nervous system, the cardiovascular system, or in the kidneys, usually require aggressive parenteral therapy requiring a critical care unit. Those hypertensive patients with severely elevated pressures but without acute end-organ effects can be aggressively managed in Cooperative Care with a variety of oral agents that can be titrated, evaluated, and changed frequently. Also, the patient can be worked up for secondary hypertension in this setting. The frequent recording of the blood pressures in Cooperative Care, may give a better view of the severity of the problem than can be obtained through outpatient encounters. Appropriate educational objectives, such as lifestyle changes (diet, exercise, alcohol, and smoking cessation) may be made easily in Cooperative Care. Also, teaching the patient or care partner how to measure blood pressure may be very valuable in followup. This can be done with the usual sphygmomanometers, or by utilizing one of the many commercially available digital units.

THE PATIENT WITH COR PULMONALE

The patient who has right-sided heart failure on the basis of pulmonary disease (Cor Pulmonale) needs treatment directed toward both the heart and the lungs. Some of the usual regimens for the treatment of congestive heart failure may be utilized, with special attention directed to the unique problems of these patients, including electrolyte imbalance, sensitivity to digitalis, etc. Titration of *oxygen therapy* is very important and may require periodic blood gas determinations and/or noninvasive measurement of oxygen saturation. Continuous ambulatory oxygen therapy may be useful in selected patients, and can be implemented in Cooperative Care. Inhalational treatments to improve oxygenation and ventilation may be crucial in treating the heart failure. All of these therapies can be accomplished in the Cooperative Care setting.

THE PATIENT WITH INFECTIVE ENDOCARDITIS

Month-long intravenous therapy of infective endocarditis may be well accomplished in Cooperative Care, and follow up blood cultures, antibiotic drug levels, serial echocardiographic studies, and assessment of clinical response are easily done. Some selected patients may be able to be discharged and complete their antibiotic therapy at home with home-care-based intravenous therapy services.

THE PATIENT WITH CARDIOVASCULAR DISEASE REQUIRING NONCARDIAC SURGERY

Patients with significant cardiovascular disease who undergo major noncardiac surgery—in particular resection of an abdominal aortic aneurysm, prolonged lower extremity vascular procedures, and extensive thoracic and abdominal surgeries—are at increased risk for intra-and postoperative myocardial infarction, congestive heart failure, and cardiac rhythm disturbances. Oftentimes, careful preoperative assessment of coronary blood flow and left ventricular function, using a variety of noninvasive, and sometimes invasive, modalities is required. Based on the results of these evaluations, some patients may need operative revascularization or valvular replacement/repair, so that they may be better able to handle the stress of their planned surgery. Other patients may benefit from catheter revascularization techniques, such as PTCA or atherectomy, while the great majority of patients may benefit from optimization of their cardiac medical regimen. These preoperative interventions/investigations may effectively be done in Cooperative Care. At the other end of the spectrum, postoperative patients may benefit from fine tuning of their cardiac regimens before hospital discharge.

In sum, the full spectrum of cardiac diagnostic and treatment modalities may be modified so that the patient may benefit from the unique clinical, psychological, and social benefits of Cooperative Care.

9

MEDICAL: THE PATIENT WITH AIDS

Jeffrey B. Greene

The concept of Cooperative Care was given life at the New York University Medical Center at virtually the same time that a new and deadly disease, AIDS, was being recognized. It is highly unlikely that the early planners of Cooperative Care could have envisioned a role for their facility in the care of the very ill patients suffering with what was later to be known as AIDS. Indeed, the physicians who grappled with those first patients practiced critical care medicine in intensive care settings. The past 12 years have seen gradual changes occur in the Cooperative Care concept which has served to help it meet the demands of health care providers charged with the care of a wider range of patients. During this same period, the illness that we now call AIDS has been dramatically altered by a variety of diagnostic, therapeutic, and biologic factors. The net result has been the evolution of a novel health care delivery system serendipitously well suited to provide the mechanism by which a patient with AIDS can receive effective hospital treatment.

AIDS MEDICINE: AN EVOLVING MEDICAL SUBSPECIALTY

Practitioners charged with the care of patients with AIDS face very different challenges than did those of a decade ago. To a large extent, the early years of AIDS medicine focused on the description of the clinical syndrome and the treatment of life-threatening opportunistic infections, such as *Pneumocystis carinii* pneumonia. Because even the etiology of AIDS was unknown then, the disease was veiled by such diverse attitudes as fear, fascination, intellectual curiosity, and apocalyptic religiosity. Much knowledge has accrued since the discovery of the etiologic agent of AIDS, the human immunodeficiency virus, in 1983. In rapid succession, advances in both the basic and clinical sciences yielded important diagnostic, therapeutic, and prophylactic modalities. There can be no question as to the impact these advances had on the lives of patients suffering from AIDS, and on the clinical expression of this illness.

The most dramatic change clinicians have observed is the stage in which they see patients present with HIV infection. In the first years of the epidemic, most had advanced AIDS, Walter Reed Class IV or V, at the time of initial diagnosis. The development of a reliable serologic test for HIV infection in 1984 allowed for the identification of large numbers of people at earlier stages of their infection. Now, AIDS physicians follow large numbers of asymptomatic HIV-infected patients. This gives the caregiver the opportunity to educate his or her patients about the signs and symptoms of the many opportunistic illnesses complicating HIV infection. The net result is that patients often present very early in the course of an infection, and the subsequent treatment is more effective and better tolerated.

The incidence of certain opportunistic infections has decreased. For example, the incidence of acute *Pneumocystis carinii* pneumonia has dropped dramatically since the widespread use of antimicrobial prophylaxis. Whereas prior to 1985 80% of patients with AIDS suffered at least one episode of *pneumocystis* pneumonia, the current incidence of this complication is less than 40%. The success in the prevention of *pneumocystis* has given birth to prophylaxis regimens for other opportunistic infections, such as central nervous system toxoplasmosis, cryptococcosis, and disseminated mycobacterium avium-intracellulare.

The result of the prophylactic approach to opportunistic infections has been a shift away from pneumocystis as the most common cause for hospitalization, to the more chronic infections, such as M. avium-intracellulare, or cytomegalovirus. Additionally, patients are living longer, in part due to opportunistic infection prophylaxis, and at lower states of immune function. The average survival following a clinical diagnosis of AIDS has more than doubled since 1983, when it was only 7 months. This very positive change has nonetheless altered the natural history of the illness by resulting in an increasing incidence of non-Hodgkin's lymphoma and other neoplasms. Polypharmaceutical prophylactic antimicrobial regimens also have added drug–drug interactions, toxicity, and drug allergy to the list of admitting diagnoses of patients with AIDS.

Antiretroviral therapy was added to the practitioner's armamentarium in 1986 in the form of zidovudine (Retrovir™). Almost immediately upon its licensure, this nucleoside analog became widely used, first in patients with advanced disease, and then in individuals with asymptomatic HIV infection. The true impact of this class of antiviral therapy upon the natural history of AIDS is still being discovered. Although evidence is lacking that zidovudine actually prolongs the life of people with AIDS, numerous studies have supported the notion that it can delay the onset of clinical AIDS. The trade off, however, is cumulative survival at very low states of immune function. Patients taking zidovudine for extended periods of time have a high incidence of non Hodgkin's lymphoma. As the efficacy of antiretroviral therapy improves with the advent of newer agents and the use of combination chemotherapy, the natural history of AIDS is bound to change even more dramatically than it has to this point.

The human immunodeficiency virus has a propensity for mutational variation, which accounts for the fact that many infected persons harbor numerous strains. In addition, genetic mutation results in the "acquisition" of viral strains resistant to the nucleoside analog antiviral agents. It also is possible that highly variable genotypes alter the pathogenicity of the virus. On theoretical grounds, the HIV has the genetic machinery to evolve rapidly to become somewhat less virulent, resulting in a more chronic illness. To what extent this may have altered the natural history of AIDS over the past decade is speculative but interesting.

Patients with AIDS have access to a huge amount of research and clinical information. This can be empowering and helpful in choosing and monitoring therapies. The cascade of information may also be distressful to patients, especially when they confront the inevitability of conflicting data or proponents of "alternative" therapies. Psychological stress has escalated in parallel with the progress realized over the past decade, and patients may present with anxiety syndromes, depression, expression of premorbid personality disorders, and mania. The psychologic impact of prolonged survival witnessing the death of friends and lovers with this illness can also result in "survivor guilt."

The profile of patients with AIDS, then, continues to change toward

a more chronic illness with longer periods of clinical stability, punctu-
ated by an everincreasing number of pharmacologic interventions, and
an increase in the incidence of infections and neoplasms previously
seen only rarely.

A CRITICAL PIECE: THE PREADMISSION EVALUATION

The effectiveness of the Cooperative Care unit as a diagnostic and
therapeutic facility rests most directly on a patient's proper preadmission evaluation by the physician. Each patient should be thoroughly
examined and, when appropriate, outpatient laboratory studies should
be obtained. The purpose of the preadmission evaluation, which
should take place no more than 2 or 3 days prior to the anticipated admission date, is twofold. First, it provides the physician an opportunity
to develop an organized treatment plan, as well as the chance to discuss this plan fully with the patient.

Second, the preadmission evaluation allows the physician the opportunity to assess the appropriateness of a Cooperative Care admission.
The assessment should consider the physical, psychosocial, and clinical status of the patient. The physical assessment includes an interim
history and a directed physical examination. Altered mental status, a
history of interruption of consciousness, or advanced dementia would
preclude a patient from admission to the unit for obvious reasons. Similarly, performance-modifying symptoms, for example, severe dyspnea,
prostration, orthostasis, or sustained hyperpyrexia, would tend to
limit the clinical success in a Cooperative Care setting. The physical
exam should be directed to identify any patient with severely abnormal vital signs, orthostatic hypotension, cyanosis, a bleeding diathe-
sis, acute abdomen, cyanosis, or an exanthem suggestive of a communicable illness.

The psychosocial condition of the patient figures prominently in the
ultimate success of a Cooperative Care hospital stay. Generally speaking, the patients who have motivated themselves into taking a proac-
tive role in their own care make the best candidates. History of severe
untreated depression, suicidal ideation, active drug dependence, or
history of antisocial behavior are contraindications for Cooperative
Care. Ideally, the primary care physician will know his or her patient
well, and will be able to determine if the Cooperative Care model fits
well with the patient's demeanor.

Some patients, especially if the illness that prompts their admission
is the first manifestation of AIDS, will feel very overwhelmed by the

demands for self-responsibility. In another instance, certain patients with cosmetically significant Kaposi's sarcoma will find it difficult to navigate the communal nature of the Cooperative Care Unit.

The social situation of the patient is also of great importance. Lack of a significant other to function as a committed care partner can make the experience burdensome to patients, and place inordinate strain on fragile support systems. The physician will usually have had the opportunity to observe the interpersonal dynamics of the patient and the proposed care partners. For very ill patients, it may be important to ascertain the availability of multiple care partners. As the demands for responsibility to the patient increase, care partner "burnout" becomes a major problem. The physical health of the care partner, especially when they too are HIV-infected, may occasionally factor into the patient's hospital experience.

The clinical status of the patient must be taken into account before committing the patient to a Cooperative Care setting. This refers to the general performance status of the patient as well as the possible diagnoses for which they require admission. Generally speaking, a Karnofsky score of 40 should preclude a patient from the Cooperative Care setting. Such a degree of debilitation renders the patient at undue risk of injury, even in the presence of a fulltime care partner. Furthermore, a poor performance status might well interfere with the beneficial evacuative and educational programs which are so much a part of the Cooperative Care experience.

The admission diagnosis also needs to be carefully considered in the context of the limitations of the Cooperative Care facility. Communicable illnesses in this setting can potentially cause major nosocomial outbreaks. Patients with a respiratory illness and a chest roentgenogram that is atypical for *Pneumocystis carinii* pneumonia should have several sputum specimens negative for acid-fast bacilli prior to admission. Similarly, a vesicular eruption demands exclusion of primary varicella or varicella-zoster prior to admission. Chronic diarrheal illnesses may be managed in Cooperative Care facilities as long as the patient is continent.

The assessment of the clinical condition is also of importance to assure that the proposed diagnostic evaluation may be undertaken as planned. For example, patients admitted with the intention of performing an invasive procedure, such as liver biopsy, should be shown to be hemostatically competent prior to admission. Likewise, patients should not be admitted for elective transbronchial biopsies before assessing their degree of hypoxemia. Finally, the preadmission clinical evaluation should be directed to anticipate the likelihood of a rapid decline in condition, or a condition that cannot be adequately treated in

Cooperative Care. For example, a patient on dideoxyinosine [DDI, Videx] with upper abdominal pain should have a serum lipase and amylase drawn prior to admission to exclude pancreatitis. Other clinical harbingers of Cooperative Care-incompatible diagnoses are serious electrolyte abnormalities, diabetes insipidus, acute deep vein thrombophlebitis, pneumothorax, renal failure, hepatic failure, and absolute neutropenia. When clinically relevant, the appropriate diagnostic studies need to be done to exclude these conditions prior to admission to Cooperative Care.

The development of the treatment plan is essential to meet the ever-increasing requirements of managed-care reimbursement. Moreover, a well laid-out plan will help the physician and the patient avail themselves of the many unique services offered in the Cooperative Care Center. For some patients, this might involve a preadmission orientation and tour of the facilities. For others, educational programs might be developed specific to their individual needs. Patients with AIDS particularly benefit from classes in nutrition, pharmacology, and vascular access (for example, Hickman catheters, etc.). Additionally, nurse specialists and social workers work with physicians in identifying those patients with special needs in their respective areas. Preadmission planning also will allow the primary care physician to assemble his or her group of consultants to ensure a smooth and rapid workup. As the team is assembled before admission, operative schedules and the proper order of diagnostic studies can be organized.

COOPERATIVE CARE: THE PHYSICIAN'S PERSPECTIVE

The Cooperative Care concept has evolved to provide a hospitable and effective venue for the care of patients with AIDS. As noted in the previous section, Cooperative Care demands an intimate knowledge of the patient's physical, mental and psychosocial health on the part of the physician. This integrated involvement with the patient, and, for that matter, with the care partner(s), helps build bonds of mutual respect and trust. This provides a solid foundation on which a successful doctor–patient relationship can be nurtured, and undoubtedly improves patient compliance and outcomes.

The Cooperative Care format utilizes a unique team approach in that the patient, and not the physician, is the "leader" of this team. The physician must make appointments to see the patients, as do the nurse clinicians, nurse specialists, social workers, nutritionists, and pharmacists. The patients are almost never seen in their suites, which serve as sanctuaries from the clinical aspects of their illnesses. The Cooperative Care approach helps to focus the many different team practitioners keenly on the patient from the moment of admission to the unit. Physicians are "backed up" efficiently and confidently by the senior nurse clinicians. Because there are multiple practitioners, the patient and care partner identify the team, rather than their physician, as their clinicians. They interface with their care team for hours each day, in contrast to the 10 or 15 minutes they might spend with their physician in an acute care setting. Patients and their care partners thereby have significant indirect access to their physicians. The result of this telescoped interaction is better patient understanding of the treatment plan, better compliance, and a more positive attitude during the hospitalization.

The Cooperative Care Unit has been increasingly suitable for the diagnosis and treatment of AIDS-related illnesses. As the unit evolved, changes in policy allowed utilization of parenteral therapies, total parenteral nutrition, continuous subcutaneous and intravenous pumps for analgesia, chemotherapy, and respiratory therapy. Two-thirds of all AIDS-related admissions can be accomplished in a Cooperative Care unit. The majority of admissions to the unit (70%) are for diagnostic purposes, and the remainder require admission for initiation of therapies.

The scope of the expertise of the health care team make Cooperative Care a true multidisciplinary unit. This gives Cooperative Care a flexibility that allows the management of a wide range of conditions. The following case illustrates the therapeutic latitude afforded the physician in the treatment of patients with AIDS.

A 42-year-old woman with AIDS was admitted for the evaluation of fever and weight loss. She reported daily temperatures to 103° F. for 5 weeks and an associated ten pound weight loss. She had a history of P. carinii pneumonia 18 months earlier. The baseline CD-4 cell count was 25 cells/mm3.

Shortly before the onset of fever, the patient suffered a traumatic closed fracture of the left patella requiring a cast for 3 weeks followed by a splint.

She was admitted with a presumptive diagnosis of opportunistic infection after an outpatient evaluation was unrevealing. Early in the workup, a CAT scan of the abdomen and pelvis was performed, which revealed a questionable thrombus in the left common femoral vein. Ultrasound of the groin documented a thrombus despite absence of any clinical signs of venous obstruction. A diagnosis of chronic Left Common Femoral Thrombophlebitis secondary to splint immobilization was made and the primary care physician placed the patient on the transfer list to the acute care facility.

Upon learning of the transfer request, the nurse clinician met with the physician and the unit's nursing supervisor. The physician was unaware of the availability of continuous infusion pumps for heparin therapy. In view of the chronicity of the phlebitis, it was decided to continue to treat the patient in Cooperative Care.

Heparin therapy proceeded with two dose changes based on BID Partial Thromboplastin Times. The fevers resolved by the second day of therapy and warfarin was started on the fifth day of heparin therapy. The patient was taught about warfarin therapy in the Education Center. She was discharged four days later. On outpatient follow up, her anticoagulation status remained well controlled, and she remained afebrile.

This case exemplifies the clinical "surprises" that can lurk in the care of AIDS patients. Moreover, it illustrates the value of the provider team, the depth of the clinical capabilities of the unit, and the usefulness of patient education in determining successful therapeutic outcomes.

The physician finds Cooperative Care "user-friendly" in the care of AIDS patients. With properly selected patients, diagnostic and treatment plans should be successfully completed on the unit. Transfer rates from Cooperative Care to the acute care facility should be less than 5% for patients with AIDS diagnoses. Partly because of the pre-admission evaluation process, and partly because of the efficiency of the unit, the average length of stay for patients with AIDS is comparatively short, 4–5 days.

Cooperative Care provides an excellent staging area for the transition of continued therapies to the home care arena. Almost all of the AIDS-related opportunistic infections require indefinite maintenance therapy, many with parenteral pharmaceuticals. The Cooperative Care Education Center provides patients and care partners with the knowledge they need to ensure safe administration of therapy at home. In addition, the contracted home care nursing staff often interact with the Cooperative Care staff to share observations useful in the assessment of the patient for home care therapies. The onsite home care assessment helps patients familiarize themselves with the particular high-tech equipment they will be using once they are home, and the Cooperative Care team can reinforce this knowledge prior to discharge.

In summary, for properly selected patients with AIDS, Cooperative Care provides the physician with all the necessary tools to provide effective, safe, and well tolerated therapeutic regimens.

COOPERATIVE CARE: THE PATIENT'S PERSPECTIVE

The majority of patients admitted to the hospital enter with the expectation that their medical condition will be improved. This goal can be attained by the vast majority of AIDS patients admitted to a Cooperative Care setting. Because of the unique aspects of AIDS, patients and their care partners often have other, less clinical expectations of the system. Most prominent is the role of the care partners, not just during the admission, but following discharge.

The Cooperative Care arena virtually enlists one or more persons to assume the role of supervisor of the overall treatment plan for the patient. This crucial task, the assignment of a partner in care, may have been one the patient was unwilling or unable to assume. The net effect is to solidify the support systems that will be operative after the patient is discharged from the hospital. The central importance of the support system becomes increasingly realized as the illness progresses. Further, because patients with AIDS often require multiple admissions to the unit over time, the opportunity exists for the patient and hospital staff to reevaluate the appropriateness of specific caregivers.

It is not unusual for a care partner to become increasingly uncomfortable in his or her role as the patient deteriorates. For some, the uneasiness may take the form of concern over contagious diseases, or their own failing health. For others, the psychological burden of caring for a terminally ill patient is too much to bear. The Cooperative Care system can quickly identify such problems by allowing the professional health care providers at all levels to observe directly the interpersonal dynamics of patient and care partner. This allows the staff to help the patient in the identification and enlistment of alternative caregivers in preparation for discharge.

Support systems for patients with AIDS extend far beyond the care partner. In some cases family members previously disenfranchised from involvement in the patient's illness can reconnect to the support network through the Cooperative Care staff. It can be extremely rewarding for patient and staff to observe a parent or sibling to regain the ability to communicate love and respect for the patient. Such experiences undoubtedly impact positively on the patient's remaining life.

Other patients also form an important part of the support systems. The community areas of the Cooperative Care Unit, such as the treatment floor, the cafeteria, and the recreation center, serve as informal meeting places for individuals so inclined. Acquaintances bred by a stay in Cooperative Care often bloom into lasting friendships. Patients will compare diagnoses and treatment schemes, and this allows them the chance to explore their illnesses with others at their own level. The reinforcement that patients can bring to bear on one another is a very positive factor in patient compliance and confidence.

Finally, the Cooperative Care staff functions in the support network long after the patient is discharged from the hospital. Nurse-clinicians, the AIDS nurse specialist, social workers, and even the nutritionists maintain important lines of communication with the patient and care partner. Frequently, one of the Cooperative Care professionals will be the one to convey a change in condition to the primary care physician of an AIDS patient at home. The sense of teamwork makes the patient feel less anxious, and enhances clinical outcomes by encouraging followup and compliance. The patient may choose to express certain feelings to a nurse or a social worker rather than to the physician. The effective increase in access to the physician helps greatly in patient management.

The Cooperative Care facility provides essential educational tools to the patient and care partner. Knowledge about pathogenesis, antimicrobials, drug–drug interactions, venous access devices, and nutrition, just to name a few areas, is empowering to the patients and makes them active participants in their care. A receptive physician can learn a great deal from motivated patients who take responsibility for their own therapies. The education process also is helpful in preparing the patient for complex home therapies. The well-instructed patient has fewer missed doses and fewer treatment mishaps, because he or she can recognize potential problems.

The indignity of AIDS for young men and women cannot be overstated. A Cooperative Care setting allows the patient privacy, quality time with family and loved ones, and superb care in a collegial, nonsterile environment. One patient recently stated when facing the prospect of hospitalization and given the choice of Cooperative Care or the acute care hospital, "Cooperative Care, of course; I don't have much time left and I don't plan to waste it in the hospital!"

COOPERATIVE CARE PITFALLS FOR THE PHYSICIAN

The most significant pitfall for the physician is improper selection of patients. Experienced AIDS practitioners can usually anticipate the degree and pace of a patient's illness quite accurately. The unit is unable to provide very frequent vital signs, blood transfusions in the patient rooms, intensive neurologic or psychiatric nursing, or continuous intravenous hydration therapy. A patient who is admitted and requires these therapies might need transfer to the traditional hospital setting. Of course, some patients will unexpectedly deteriorate during their Cooperative Care stay and require transfer.

Another problem for some patients stems from the communal nature of Cooperative Care. For example, a patient admitted to the unit for a first episode of *Pneumocystis carinii* pneumonia might be terrified to see first-hand other AIDS patients who are much farther along in their illnesses. Time and sensitivity on the part of many members of the Cooperative Care team are needed to alleviate the fears and anxieties of these patients. The communal atmosphere would probably not be appropriate for individuals who have high public recognition and wish to keep their medical problems a secret. The interaction between patients and care partners also presents a problem in cases of previously unrecognized personality disorders. A disruptive patient or care partner can impact on the care of many patients. Such individuals require urgent transfer off the unit.

The physician should be prepared to defend his or her treatment or diagnostic plan to any patient entering the Cooperative Care facility. Motivated patients will use the hospital experience to further their knowledge and satisfy their curiosities about the appropriateness of their own treatment. Although not precisely a pitfall, the physician should anticipate a potentially animated discussion comparing different approaches to the same clinical problem.

CONCLUSION

Cooperative Care is a concept of health care delivery that works brilliantly for many patients with AIDS. It embraces the objectives of self-empowerment through education and independence. The Cooperative Care experience builds the support system networks that are so essential to AIDS patients as their illness progresses, and helps bridge clinical care into the home after discharge. A wide spectrum of disease states may be diagnosed and treated effectively in the Cooperative Care setting when proper preadmission evaluations are undertaken. As the costs of health care for patients with AIDS continue to soar, Cooperative Care facilities may prove to be a more effective, lower-cost alternative to traditional acute care hospitalization.

The wedding may be over, but the marriage of this unique health care delivery system and the evolving clinical science of AIDS medicine is likely to remain vital well into the 21st century.

10

MEDICAL: THE PATIENT WITH MALIGNANCY

James L. Speyer

There have been major technological advances and successes in the treatment of malignancy in recent years. But in addition to precise diagnosis and effective treatment, cancer patients feel the need, more than most patients with other types of diseases, for a system in which they can regain some control over their own lives. To regain control, they reach out to a wide variety of resources. To the extent possible, it helps, too, to permit the patient to actually participate in elements of their cancer care.

The family of the cancer patient undergoes much the same feeling of loss of control. Family members frequently express their sense of impotence, not knowing how to or not being able to help the patient. The patient is the epicenter of a complex set of psychosocial relationships that have a forceful impact on their care. It is the power of this pointed focus on the sick cancer patient that needs to be harnessed by the professionals and channelled into productive avenues. Involving the family in care, and supporting that involvement with in-depth education, is the solution to maximizing the support available to each patient.

The Cooperative Care setting meets these needs ideally. It stimulates patients to remain as physically active as they can tolerate and discourages, but does not prohibit, them from assuming the "sick" role. The requirement that the patient, with the aid of the care partner, come to the centralized therapeutic center, education center and dining room enforces ambulation, or at least mobility. The patient's activity level in Cooperative Care more closely resembles a normal existence than the constricted daily pattern of activity expected on a traditional medical unit. Taking meals at a table with other people is much closer to a healthy pattern of life than is eating in bed or sitting on the edge of a bed. Being permitted to wear street clothes if desired, rather than a hospital gown, enhances self-image. Taken together, these seemingly small facets of behavior empower patients who are struggling to place their illness in some sort of understandable context, enabling them to come closer to living with the cancer rather than having it overwhelm them with a sense of helpless inactivity and futility.

Giving patients a share in the responsibility for their own care helps to give them back some control over life. Small details count toward returning dignity to patients. For example, it helps to have them share in planning the timing of appointments. It helps to have patients sense the importance of reporting symptoms. It helps to have patients handle their own medications. It helps to have them work with the oncology nurse specialists to modify their treatment plan and symptom management.

Involving the family and close friends as care partners empowers them as well. Their frustration in watching a loved one with cancer is alleviated by including them in the process of caring for the patient. Although pushing a patient in a wheelchair to attend an appointment with the nurse or physician may seem a small step to some, it is a concrete demonstration of the care partner's dedication and sacrifice for the patient's welfare. Calling the nurse when the patient feels poorly and administering and recording medication also helps the family member to feel what is true: that he or she is an essential part of the health care team. Enhancing this positive feeling helps to alleviate some of the potential for impatience and despair. It also sets up a pattern that can lead to a collaborative relationship both in Cooperative Care and later at home. The mutual collaboration and familiarity with details of treatment also serves to alleviate anxiety both for the patient and the family.

ONCOLOGY NURSE SPECIALISTS

Oncology nurse specialists are the main providers of many of the services for cancer patients in a focused environment. They bring their high degree of advanced training and specialized knowledge to the care of these people. Their extensive clinical experience with cancer patients in Cooperative Care provides a clearly delineated focus for cancer care. The oncology nurse specialist's first-hand knowledge of the evolution of signs and symptoms, and of the patient's appearance and tolerance of treatments from visit to visit, is invaluable.

The oncology nurse specialist also represents continuity of care for patients who undergo multiple-day hospitalizations or repeated admissions. This continuity, in addition to that of the physician, provides a core of cancer-related care with much greater depth than would be the case if the continuity were maintained by one professional alone. This constancy of caregiving personnel adds greatly to the comfort of the patient and family. The oncology nurse specialist comes to know and understand the likes, dislikes, and quirks of the patient and the family, as well as their level of sophistication in understanding the diagnosis and prognosis, all of which helps in planning care for them. An oncology nurse specialist who knows the patient well often is the first to appreciate subtle changes in the patient's clinical status or emotional state, before they become apparent to others.

In Cooperative Care, instead of limiting the diagnostic spectrum, an identified group of oncology-specific professionals within the unit define the focus and meet the needs of these patients, even though the unit as a whole handles a broad spectrum of diagnoses. This works, in part, because of the large number of patients with malignancy in Cooperative Care, who represent approximately 20% of the volume of the unit. The frequency with which oncology problems are faced by the staff as a whole, combined by the support provided by the expertise of the oncology nurse specialists, has raised the cancer-related skills of the entire professional group well above that found on most general medical units. As a result of these factors, the nurse-educators, nurse-clinicians, social workers, pharmacists and nutritionists in Cooperative Care have become strongly motivated to acquire the extra knowledge they need to become valuable assets in the plan of care for these patients.

EXAMPLES OF TREATMENT PROTOCOLS

In order for patients to be admitted to Cooperative Care, they must meet the criteria for hospitalization that are valid for traditional hospital units. The therapy and diagnostic procedures to be performed must be of such a nature that they are not regularly provided on an outpatient basis. Some of these therapies warrant admission by virtue of their duration: for example, treatment with ifosphamide combined with mesna, with cisplatin requiring prolonged intravenous hydration, prolonged infusion of 5–fluorouracil, or 24-hour infusion of taxol. Other treatment regimens that might require admission include multi drug treatments of long duration, such as the combination of DTIC/BCNU/Cisplatin, some multiple-day treatment protocols, or a prolonged antiemetic schedule with intravenous odantseran.

Patients undergoing combined modality treatment, such as those with small-cell lung cancer receiving twice-daily radiation therapy in conjunction with chemotherapy, require hospitalization because such a regimen is impractical on an outpatient basis. In addition to admission prompted by a specific treatment regimen, other patients require hospitalization because of disability resulting from extreme debilitation and weakness. Others require admission because close observation is needed while, for example, they are undergoing pain control management, perhaps in conjunction with radiation therapy or chemotherapy.

Although these patients require inpatient care, many of them are not totally bedbound. If, for example, a patient is receiving chemotherapy containing cisplatinum for 4 hours, pretherapy and posttherapy intravenous hydration, and antiemetics, the infusions can be delivered while the patient is sitting in a lounge chair. The patient then returns to his or her room and later, if able to eat, comes to the dining room for a meal. Concurrent administration of intravenous antibiotics, analgesics, and other treatments can be handled in a similar fashion.

A problem faced by many cancer patients is repeated venipuncture and repeated intravenous infusions, with scarring from sclerosing agents culminating in limited venous access. Because many chemotherapeutic regimens require that reliable intravenous access be available, surgically implanted access ports, such as mediports or Hickman catheters, are commonly needed. Learning how to deal with a venous access port is one of the goals of the educational program at Cooperative Care.

Long-duration infusions are simplified by using a portable infusion pump, permitting the patient to remain mobile during the course of the chemotherapy. Some of the chemotherapeutic regimens which are amenable to this technique are the 72-hour infusion of 5–fluorouracil, the 96-hour infusion of adriamycin, the 24-hour infusion of taxol, and the investigational 21-day infusion of topotecan. Of course, the portable infusion pump also is useful for administration of total parenteral nutrition.

Although portable intravenous infusion pumps have permitted some patients to be treated entirely on an outpatient basis, some still require inpatient care because of concurrent therapies, complications, or other reasons for close observation, as discussed earlier.

An advantage to combining the use of a portable infusion pump with the Cooperative Care setting is that patients are able to maintain some feeling of independence and control while having ready access to all the hospital services they need. Using a portable infusion pump, physical activity can be continued, rather than having the individual degraded to a sedentary level or forced to be confined to unneeded bed rest.

OTHER PATIENT SERVICES

In addition to the clinical services discussed so far, the service provided by the Cooperative Care Education Center completes the comprehensive approach to the management of the cancer patient. Education related to the diagnosis and treatment is part of this, of course. Equally important is attention to psychosocial needs. This includes individualized assistance in dealing with critical problems, helping both the patient and family cope with the disease and its aftermath, arranging assistance with transportation, guidance with finances, and direction in implementing a home care plan. The individualized help is fortified by support group sessions in which a social worker, perhaps in conjunction with a nurse-educator, can facilitate transference of insights from one patient and family to another. The collaborative environment of Cooperative Care provides an ideal setting in which this can happen.

Nutritionists in the education center provide specialized instruction in dietary modification and nutritional support for cancer patients. This might include special diets for patients who experience difficulty swallowing, the use of nutritional supplements, or the initiation of tube feedings or even total parenteral nutrition. Calorie counts and daily weight measurements with blood chemistry confirmation are easily accomplished. The ability to have the nutritionists in Cooperative Care monitor patients who are using the dining room for their meals provides a closer approximation to what would be happening later at home. This in itself often leads to better detection of nutritional problems and a better outcome for patients, including a decrease in the rate of readmission for those problems which can be intercepted.

Since many cancer patients are on complicated drug regimens, and face many potential or actual side effects and interactions, the services of the Education Center pharmacist are vitally important. Educating patients and their families about individual drugs decreases anxiety and increases compliance. Gaining a fuller understanding of the expected side effects not only eases the patient's mind, but also alerts both patient and family to those questions which might arise later at home. Thus, they will be better prepared to recognize medication-related problems and to report them to the physician when they occur.

In preparation for management at home, pharmacists, nurse-educators, nurse-clinicians, and oncology nurse specialists teach patients and their care partners how to reconstitute and self-administer parenteral medications. Among the drugs that are likely to be self-administered at home are insulin, granulocyte colony stimulating factor (GCSF), granulocyte-macrophage colony stimulating factor (GMCSF), erythropoietin, interferon, and interleukin-2, as well as investigational drugs such as interleukin-3, interleukin-4, macrophage colony stimulating factor (MCSF), and PIXY-321.

Pain control services are particularly relevant to cancer patients. Keeping the patient as mobile as possible is best, as it does little good to control pain while the individual is confined to bed, only to send him or her home to a more active existence in which the pain is not well controlled at all. Cooperative Care is an ideal environment for realistically adjusting the pain control regimen to the patient's later outpatient requirements, whether by oral medications, transdermal drugs, parenteral agents via subcutaneous injection, or an intravenous infusion pump.

The comprehensive approach to diagnosis and treatment, so important to the cancer patient, is clearly provided by the Cooperative Care setting. Diagnostic testing, consultations, education, and therapy are carried out in the constant presence of the family support system. In addition, the newly diagnosed patient in particular benefits from observing and interacting with patients who have been receiving treatment for a longer period of time. New patients and their family members rapidly learn by example, from those who have had longer first-hand experience, how to live with the illness rather than be controlled by it. The multidisciplinary professional team, coupled with active involvement of the family or friend care partner, brings it all together. Encouraging the patient's and family's behavior pattern to be more like that at home, yet providing all the supports of a focused environment for dealing with malignancy, Cooperative Care is a most humane cancer center.

11

THE NURSING PERSPECTIVE

Kimberly S. Glassman, Jeanne Dzurenko, and
Alan R. Schukman

BEDSIDE CARE VS. CENTRALIZED SERVICES

The patient-centered care movement has caused major restructuring
of nursing units and of the traditional ways in which hospital care is
delivered. Most efforts in this movement, however, have been directed
toward developing and utilizing a multiskilled worker and minimizing
"inconvenience" to patients by bringing more decentralized clinical
services directly to the patient's bedside or nursing unit. For example,
laboratory services, electrocardiography, physiotherapy and, in some
instances, radiology, are advocated for bedside delivery on those units
(Brider, 1992; O'Malley & Serpico-Thompson, 1992; Watson,
Shortridge, Jones, Rees, & Stephens, 1991).

Cooperative Care chose a different route in 1979. Instead of delivering all these clinical services to the patient's bedside, thus encouraging further immobility, it was proposed that in Cooperative Care the
patient come to centralized clinical, educational and dining services.

In addition, instead of cultivating a hospital employee who would act as a multi skilled worker, Cooperative Care was centered on the use of a family member or friend who would become actively involved in assisting, caring for, and learning about the patient's needs and treatments.

ADVANCED NURSING PRACTICE

In an academic medical center, a non teaching unit or, in other words, any patient care unit that functions in the absence of house staff, can create unique opportunities for experienced nursing staff. The Cooperative Care Unit created just such an advanced nursing practice opportunity for senior registered nurses at NYU Medical Center.

In order for it to function as an advanced nursing practice unit, Cooperative Care has employed only nurses who meet the minimum requirements of having a baccalaureate degree and 3 to 5 years of acute care medical/surgical nursing experience. In actual fact, the majority of the nurses in Cooperative Care are Master's-prepared, and the staff has an average of 11 years of experience in nursing.

Of course, a major focus of nursing in Cooperative Care is on identifying each patient's educational needs so that they can participate in their own care, along with the care partner and professionals. In order for the nursing staff to fully provide patients with the skills and techniques needed to provide such care, it was thought that a professional nurse at a higher level of practice would be needed.

NURSING STAFF RATIOS AND SCHEDULING

As of this writing, there are 33 full-time equivalents (FTE's) for clinical registered nurse positions in the Therapeutic Center of Cooperative Care. This total has risen periodically in order to provide care to the rising patient acuity level as the years progressed, just as patient acuity level has risen during that same period in hospitals throughout the country. One-third of the current number of nurses staffed the unit when it opened in 1979.

At present, clinical nurses care for approximately 13 to 15 patients each on the day and evening shifts, with night shift nurses (from 12 midnight to 8 A.M.) carrying a patient load of 34 to 35 patients each. Nurses are assigned to the unit 24 hours a day, and are responsible for making their professional clinical observations and treatments, for overseeing the care partners' participation, and for determining what and when to report to the attending physicians.

Patients with a wide variety of medical diagnoses are managed in Cooperative Care. The nurse who can perform as a comprehensively skilled generalist, rather than as a limited-scope specialist, has the greater stature in the Cooperative Care setting.

Flexible scheduling to meet the needs of the mature professional has helped make Cooperative Care a nursing unit with one of the lowest rates of turnover in the Medical Center. A combination of traditional 8-hour shifts and flex-time 12-hour shifts has allowed 24-hour coverage, with the heaviest concentration of staffing from 8 A.M. to 8 P.M., Sunday through Thursday, with lower staffing on weekends. Experienced nurses were paired with one another to cover a number of shifts per week and to participate in self-scheduling. This helped to ensure a primary nursing focus and limited pairs of nurses, even with flex-time scheduling. For example, the nurse pairs are either 8 hours on days and evenings or 12 hours on days, caring for their team of patients. This combination of traditional and flex-time scheduling has allowed better coverage at peak work hours. Some flex-time pairs have worked together for years, and have proven to be an exception to the argument that flex-time shifts fragment and impede continuity of care.

The management team consists of a clinical director, a head nurse (with 24–hour responsibility), and an evening/night clinical coordinator. The original team, while differently configured, had the opportunity to create a unit from "scratch," learning along the way. As the largest patient care unit of Tisch Hospital, Cooperative Care is governed by the general nursing department policies and procedures, yet because of its uniqueness, it is often the exception. At NYU Medical Center, many policies are set to gradually increase the scope of a nurse's responsibility as he or she progresses up the clinical ladder. With patient safety as a number one concern, employing nurses at the top of the clinical ladder mitigates the need for the degree of supervision required for less-experienced staff.

Policies in Cooperative Care are "written in pencil" because they change hourly, due to constant refinement from "what works best" to "what works best for this patient/care partner now." While they are better able to work in a "flexible" environment, experienced staff still express the need for some ground rules.

In addition, due to the collaborative nature of nursing practice in Cooperative Care, many of the early patient care scenarios played out in the following manner. A patient arrives in the Education Center with a supportive care partner; is well prepared for a Cooperative Care admission by the physician; is brought medications, and pre-admission orders are in. However, this best-case scenario has rarely occurred in 15 years. Thus, nurses have quickly learned to adapt the system to meet needs of individual patients. The patient who "rolled" into the Education Center on a stretcher in a body cast, was in fact, able to be cut out of his cast by his orthopedic surgeon prior to leaving the Education Center. The patient who arrives via ambulance on a nitroglycerin drip is immediately sent to the Observation Unit.

Initially, patients requiring nursing intervention every 4 hours or less were the rule for Cooperative Care. Now, patients receive intermittent IV medication around the clock. The use of some "home care like" devices (small, portable infusion pumps) helps to eliminate some nursing visits. It can be difficult for a patient to travel to the 14th floor every 1–2 hours for a variety of IV medications and treatments. Sometimes these patients remain in the Observation Unit, or "camp out" on the 14th floor for the day. Sometimes they must be transferred to Tisch Hospital.

Early in the unit's history, patients who presented with acute illness on admission (temperature 106, hypotension, chest pain, shortness of breath) were redirected to the Emergency Room for stabilization and admission to the traditional hospital. Due to overcapacity of both the Emergency Room and hospital beds, these patients are now stabilized in Cooperative Care.

Using the postprocedure recovery room as the acute holding area has advantages and disadvantages. Certainly, the traditional acute set up lends itself to easy management of the patient with emergent needs. However, it also requires you to find a different space for recovery. Cooperative Care uses examination rooms, which in turn can impact negatively on the ability to see routine patients. Learn from our mistakes.

ENCOURAGING PATIENT AND CARE PARTNER INDEPENDENCE

One of the more challenging aspects of nursing in this setting is cultivating each nurse's ability to stimulate the patient and care partner to act somewhat independently, participating in their care and making observations while in their room together. This is dramatically different from the focus of nurses in a traditional setting, where they are accustomed to "doing for" each patient. Instead, in Cooperative Care, an opportunity is provided for the patient to perform the task, if previously taught, or to observe the nurse, and to progressively develop independence in performing the task. Although some errors are inevitable, it is considered preferable that errors by the patient and care partner occur while both are still in the Cooperative Care setting. There, the professionals are available for advice and intervention 24-hours a day.

Much of the nursing care delivered in Cooperative Care is carried out through the actions of others. Although it sounds like circular reasoning, encouraging the active participation of patients and their families or significant others is key to their successful learning, just as learning is key to their successful participation. In other words, if the need for learning is felt by the patient/care partner team, they will be ripe for learning, and the knowledge gleaned can effectively be put into action.

The teaching can be done via a combination of observation and supervision by the clinical nursing staff in the Therapeutic Center and by the educational staff in the Education Center. Following the training sessions, the patient and care partner perform the task independently in their room, and thus become truly prepared for continuing their care fully independently following discharge.

The physical separation of the living quarters for the patient and care partner from the centralized clinical services helps to promote patient independence by keeping the nurse partly in the role of coach and advisor, rather than entirely a controlling "do-er." The patient and care partner can attempt solutions much as they do at home, but in Cooperative Care they have the assistance of a nurse who can individually tailor strategies to meet their needs. This works much better than relying on the traditional "hospital procedure," without individual adaptation, as that might be difficult for the patient and care partner to follow at home.

Much care was taken initially to distinguish between those tasks that require professionals and those for which the patient and care partner should be responsible, both in Cooperative Care and later at home. In general, the "low-tech" tasks, such as attention to personal hygiene, feeding, maintaining mobility and administration of oral medications, are relegated almost exclusively to the care partner, while "high-tech" tasks, such as administering intravenous infusions, blood transfusions, and the like are the province of the professional nursing staff. Today, however, more and more inpatient care has become high-tech. This presents new challenges to patients, care partners, and nurses alike. Multiple intravenous medications are infused via a Hickman catheter, total parenteral nutrition commonly is needed, and self-injection of a variety of medications is now commonplace. The same educational process of observing professionals as a start, then progressively transferring each task to the patient/care

partner team, is applied to handling these issues, as is the case with
more mundane tasks.

NURSE SPECIALISTS

In addition to the generalists, clinical nurse specialists historically
have played a role in the Cooperative Care Unit. As the complexity of
inpatient oncology regimens increased, a total of four full-time equiva-
lent oncology nurse specialists were hired to provide specialized education, administer chemotherapy, and handle symptom management.
The oncology nurse-educators and nurse clinicians provide orientation
to the Cooperative Care environment and more general clinical nursing care for those patients. An AIDS clinical nurse specialist position
was added in 1989 in order to meet the needs of the rising HIV-positive
patient population, with their intricate problems. An AIDS social
work position, specifically addressing the needs of the HIV patient,
was added in 1990 to enhance the support of these people and their
care partners, and to provide more comprehensive care via an AIDS
team approach.

NURSING ATTENDANTS

Nursing attendants and clerical staff complete the nursing staffing in
Cooperative Care. Nursing attendants (8.6 FTEs) assist the professional nurses in managing the larger patient/nurse ratio by tracking
each nurse's patient appointments, obtaining vital signs and daily
weights, and assisting with bedside care while the patient is in the observation unit. Clerical staff (eleven FTEs) handle the large volume of
computerized patient record documents, and assist in admission functions and scheduling of tests and procedures.

THE OBSERVATION UNIT

The Observation Unit, a six-bed postprocedure recovery area, is staffed
by two registered nurses from 8:30 A.M. until 8:30 P.M., with peak
staffing in the afternoon and evening. These nurses are responsible for
providing bedside care for and observation of postprocedure patients,
and for assisting in reinforcing the postprocedure information required before patients and care partners can be released to a more
semi-independent existence in their own room. As the care partner is

present during the patient's observation unit stay, the nurse can ascertain that the care partner is competent and confident in such techniques as recording intake and output, checking pulses, registering the color of the extremities, and noting the presence of sensation and motor function following invasive vascular procedures. The care partner is thoroughly instructed as to when and why to call the nurse for help.

The observation unit also serves as a "holding area" for those patients who are deemed temporarily too unstable to return to their room with a care partner. Traditional bedside nursing care then is provided in the observation unit until the crisis abates or transfer to the Intensive Care Unit is arranged.

PATIENT SCHEDULES

Patients receive a daily schedule indicating the various appointments for education, clinical care, X-rays, and blood tests. Medical visits are usually arranged directly with the patients by their personal physician, and take place either in the Therapeutic Center or in the patient's room. Diagnostic tests are scheduled on a daily basis, but may not be indicated at a specific time in the patient schedule, due to the "on-call" nature of many of the tests.

The professional staff view the patient's schedule and arrange their plan of care accordingly. Each nurse schedules his or her appointments throughout the shift, while considering the patient and care partner's individual needs. Each patient is given at least a daily appointment which includes a complete physical assessment, in addition to any scheduled treatments. At that session, the nurse discusses with the patient and care partner how they are coping with their aspects of care, particularly with self-administration of medication.

Subsequent appointments are scheduled throughout the day and evening for further doses of intravenous medications, and for observation of self-injection or dressing techniques after the patient has attended the relevant Education Center class. Regularly scheduled meetings among the members of the professional team ensure that the progress of the patient and care partner is on target for discharge.

CONCLUSION

Overall, Cooperative Care provides all traditional care, but it is delivered in a unique format. Each patient contact is focused on the patient/care partner team's competence in hospital and their readiness for discharge. The emphasis is continually on learning. Clinical tasks initially might take longer than in a traditional medical/surgical nursing unit, as they are performed with an "audience." The "audience" often is insecure initially regarding their ability to manage the task, thus the setting encourages and stimulates their relatively rapid and progressive evolution from "watcher" to "do-er." After the patient and care partner become competent, they in effect begin to multiply the nurse's efforts, so that the clinical tasks are then being performed more rapidly than the nursing staff alone would have been able to perform them, since many more hands are involved. The nurse's role here is not only that of clinician, but also that of teacher and coach, continually adapting the hospital routine to future home needs.

12

EDUCATION

Grace Phelan and Shirley A. Garnett

CENTRAL ROLE OF EDUCATION

The philosophy of Cooperative Care is based on the premise that patients have the right to participate as full partners in their care. A strong and comprehensive health educational program is essential for the patient and care partner to attain the knowledge and skills needed for them to fully and effectively participate in their management during Cooperative Care hospitalization. Thus, the educational process is central to the success of Cooperative Care, and opportunities for learning and evaluation have been built in and actually permeate the entire period of hospitalization.

Of course, education begins prior to admission, with the actions of physicians and their office staff orienting patients and care partners so that they will know what to expect about the philosophy of Cooperative Care and its physical environment when they arrive. Patients and care partners with questions are encouraged to contact the Education Center and speak with the appropriate health professional even before arrangements for admission have been confirmed. Patients who are in traditional nursing units of Tisch Hospital and who are anticipating that they will be transferred to Cooperative Care are encouraged to view an orientation video of Cooperative Care on one of the medical center-wide patient education Closed Circuit television channels. Printed materials that describe the unit also are available, both for patients who already are in Tisch Hospital and for patients in their physician's offices.

As hospital lengths of stay have become shorter, with elimination of many preoperative days, pre admission testing has become more commonplace. This has created a new opportunity for patient and care partner education, as well as orientation. Among the questions that frequently are asked during the pre admission testing session are: "What is going to happen to us?" and "What will I, as the care partner, be asked to do?"

Having a nurse-educator answer these and other related questions, as well as allowing the patient and care partner to voice their concerns can go a long way in helping to alleviate the predictable pre admission anxiety.

Because patient education is so essential to the functioning of Cooperative Care, the unit has had, from its inception, a large area identified as an educational center, with its own specifically designated staff, equipment and materials to facilitate this function.

The Education Center is staffed by a multidisciplinary team consisting of nurse-educators, nutritionists, pharmacists, social workers, a movement/relaxation therapist, and support personnel.

THE NURSE-EDUCATOR

Nurse-educators are registered nurses who have Master's Degrees in Education and at least 3 to 5 years of medical/surgical nursing experience. Their primary functions are to assess patients' and care partners' educational needs, to plan and implement an appropriate program to meet those needs, and to evaluate the patient and care partner response to the education program and the treatment regimen.

Generally, the nurse-educator is the first health professional whom the patient and care partner meet upon their arrival at Cooperative Care. After viewing an orientation video, the patient and care partner are interviewed by a nurse-educator. During that initial session, the nurse-educator ascertains the patient's reason for hospitalization, reviews the present illness and past medical history, confirms the care partner's availability and appropriateness, and assesses the patient's and care partner's educational needs.

Together the patient, care partner, and nurse-educator discuss what educational needs exist and plan appropriate interventions. Some teaching takes place at this initial session. Examples of the topics which are addressed at this introductory meeting include: a review of the signs and symptoms for which the nurse-clinician in the therapeutic center should be contacted, what to do to obtain help in an emergency, and how to safely use a wheelchair. The patient and care partner are scheduled for more in-depth matters later, and also are advised of the scope of educational programs which are available to them during their stay. In addition, they are introduced to the program of self-administration of medication (see below).

The nurse-educator conducts individual or group classes on a wide variety of topics. Examples of topics which are frequently covered are: "After coronary bypass surgery," "Total parenteral nutrition," and "Sick-day rules if you are taking insulin."

Information and teaching techniques are tailored to the individual patient's needs, taking into account any recognized factors that may have an impact on learning, such as the patient's age, any impairment of hearing or vision, the formal educational background, the presence of pain or discomfort, or undue anxiety.

Educational sessions might be one-on-one, the nurse-educator dealing with a single patient and his or her care partner or groups with several patients and their care partners. Group sessions are preferred whenever feasible, both because they use staff time more efficiently, and because they promote patient and care partner support by sharing the experiences and questions of others.

GENERALISTS VS. SPECIALIST EDUCATORS

A key decision that was faced when the education center was being developed was whether to hire professionals, who had specialized clinical expertise, or generalists, who had broad experience and who could deal with a variety of medical conditions. NYU Medical Center's Cooperative Care Unit decided that, at least for the Education Center, the "generalists" route would be the best option. A professional staff with solid seasoning and wide experience, as well as advanced degrees, was considered the essential ingredient.

Lesson outlines, in-service courses, staff conferences and handouts have been prepared, and are continually being developed, to ensure that the educational staff has a good overview of the most commonly encountered conditions. The staff includes resource people with particular expertise, including clinical nurse specialists, who act as experts for specific issues when referrals are needed. As previously mentioned, there are specialists in oncology and AIDS.

Individual staff members are encouraged to expand their knowledge and expertise in their specific areas of interest. For example, one nurse-educator who has done extensive reading and research on diabetes acts as a resource person to the staff, available to help them deal with the more complex, intricate problems. A nutritionist who has had extensive experience with total parenteral nutrition assists the other nutritionists, who had less experience, when total parenteral nutrition patients were first introduced. Now, of course, all the Cooperative Care nutritionists are responsible for handling patients undergoing total parenteral nutrition.

This generalist approach may not work for every institution. If an institution consists mostly of subspecialty units, then a "specialist" approach may be the better option.

THE NUTRITIONIST

Cooperative Care nutritionists are registered dieticians who have at least 3 to 5 years of experience and have either a Master's Degree or have completed a 1-year internship in addition to their work experience.

Referrals for nutrition counseling can arise as requests from the physician, the nurse-clinician, the patient or the care partner. In addition, a self-administered assessment form helps to identify patients who may have eating problems, such as anorexia, nausea, vomiting, and diarrhea, as well as those who are on modified diets.

A typical nutrition counseling session consists of three components. These are: 1) effecting a nutritional assessment of the patient, looking at a typical day's food and fluid intake; 2) formulating a plan of intervention to address the patient's specific needs; and 3) outlining a strategy for subsequent evaluation. Counseling related to very complex dietary regimens usually takes place over a few days, allowing time for the patient to assimilate information at his or her own pace. Props are used, at times, to help counseling. The props involve the use of food models to teach portion size, nutrition labels to help decode them, restaurant menus and "what if" situations. Emphasis is placed on the changes the patient is able to make.

Of course, in addition to participating in these formal educational sessions, the patient actually puts the assimilated knowledge directly into practice in the dining room at each mealtime. Thus, the nutritionist looks on each meal as an active participation educational opportunity, as though it were a practical examination.

In practice, a nutritionist is available at lunchtime to answer questions and to help the patient make appropriate selections. This actually is a great advantage, as it facilitates the nutritionist's ability to identify problems with understanding or compliance. If the patient is truly going to be noncompliant with, or intolerant of, the prescribed diet, then alterations might be necessary in the dosage of medications, such as insulin or diuretics. These dosages can be more realistically titrated for the patient's home situation than they can be in a traditional hospital unit.

THE PHARMACIST AND SELF-ADMINISTRATION OF MEDICATION

One of the unique aspects of Cooperative Care is the Self-Administration of Medication (SAM) program. This component of Cooperative Care grew out of the philosophy that patients have the right to participate fully in their care, and that a strong education program is essential to give the patient and care partner the knowledge required for this to happen. The goal of the SAM program is that the patient and care partner will be able to accurately administer all the patient's medication prior to discharge.

The key players of the SAM program are the patient, the care partner, the nurse-clinician in the Therapeutic Center, the nurse-educator, and the Education Center pharmacist. At the time of admission, the nurse-educator briefly assesses the patient's level of understanding about each of his or her drugs. Questions asked include: Does the patient know the names of each drug? Why are they being taken? How often are they needed per day? Are the medications being taken as prescribed? The nurse-educator describes the SAM program to the patient and care partner, explaining the goal. The medications are then discussed, and the patient is given written information sheets that describe each drug. The nurse-educator then schedules an individual educational session with the pharmacist for the patient and care partner on the following day.

At the time of the initial clinical assessment in the therapeutic center, the nurse-clinician develops a schedule, in consultation with the patient, of when to take his or her medications. The Cooperative Care medication administration schedule differs somewhat from the scheduled times of administration of the same drugs on the medical/surgical nursing units of the traditional part of the hospital. For example, if the patient will be taking medication four times in 24-hours, in most traditional units the drug will be administered at 6-hour intervals, even though that might mean interruption of sleep for a middle-of-the-night dose. In Cooperative Care, on the other hand, the medications usually will be administered four times during hours in which the patient is expected to be awake; namely, the first dose at awakening and the last dose at bedtime, with intervening doses at noon and in early evening. Whenever possible, staff try to utilize the timing schedule the patient was on at home to facilitate future adherence to the prescribed medication regimen.

The patient and care partner will not only be self-administering the medications, but will be recording that they have actually administered them. Two variants of a charting document have been developed in order to meet the needs of patients with different levels of understanding. The form that is most often used lists each medication by name, with the times for its administration in adjoining columns. Although this document meets the needs of most patients, some need a simpler sheet. For these people, an alternate form is available, organized by time of day, and giving the drugs which are to be taken at the specified hours. In unusual circumstances, further modifications can be made to meet individual needs; for example, the time of day can be listed with actual pills taped onto the sheet for extra clarity.

The nurse-clinician reviews the medication schedule and confirms the patient's and care partner's level of understanding. At this point, the medications might be dispensed to the patient/care partner team, in containers identical to those used for outpatients, with labels precisely like those used by outpatient pharmacies for patients at home.

At the individual teaching session with the pharmacist, the patient and care partner bring their medication schedule sheet as a starting point for further discussion. The pharmacist reviews the following information about each drug: the name of the medication; how to take it; what times to take it; whether there are any food/drug or drug/drug interactions; how the drugs should be stored; common and uncommon side effects; when to contact the physician for side effects; and other precautions. At this time, the patient and care partner also are given the opportunity to have the pharmacist answer their questions. If the patient has not yet received the medications, the pharmacist will bring them to the session and dispense them directly. As part of the pharmacist's evaluation, the patient might be asked to select from the various bottles of drugs which ones he or she will take at a specified time. After the educational session, the pharmacist makes a recommendation about the patient's ability to self-medicate. Although the pharmacist and nurse rarely disagree on their assessment of the patient and care partner's ability to self-medicate, it is the nurse-clinician in the Therapeutic Center who actually makes the final decision regarding SAM.

In some cases, a follow-up pharmacy education session is necessary. Each education session lasts approximately 20 minutes, but patients who are on numerous medications might have a session last as long as 40 minutes.

If other medications are added to the patient's treatment regimen after the pharmacy educational session has been completed, patients are given the appropriate supplemental information sheets, the information is reviewed with the patient and care partner by the nurse-clinician, and a telephone or in-person additional session with the pharmacist may be arranged. Of course, the medication administration schedule sheet is appropriately revised.

Patients are advised to bring their medication schedule sheets with them to all nursing appointments, so that accuracy of medication administration and charting can be reviewed regularly, and so that the depth of understanding can be periodically reassessed.

THE SOCIAL WORKER

The role of the social worker at Cooperative Care combines the two functions of discharge planning and counseling. When Cooperative Care initially opened, discharge plans were much less complex than they are today. Most Cooperative Care patients were sent home, with followup entirely the responsibility of their primary physician. There was an occasional referral to a home care nursing service. However, the increasing complexity of hospital care and health care has caused a major shift toward much greater emphasis on detailed discharge planning. Shortened lengths of stay have also contributed to this shift in emphasis, underscoring the importance of short-term problem solving and referral to community resources. For example, arranging for numerous "high-tech" services in the home, or for hospice services, is a commonplace need today.

The presence of the care partner, usually a family member or close friend, also provides the social worker with a unique opportunity for counseling. Issues that might not surface in a more traditional setting, and which can complicate the discharge plan, become more apparent in this setting. Support groups are a logical outgrowth of the milieu at Cooperative Care. Over the years, the focus has evolved as populations have changed. General stress management groups have given way to patient or care partner groups for targeted populations, such as those with AIDS or cancer. In addition to the formal support groups organized by the professional staff, informal support groups spring up spontaneously among various patients and care partners.

For the social worker, a key ingredient in keeping the support group viable is being flexible. Flexibility is essential in selection of the topics to be covered, as well as in choosing the time of the sessions. The social worker must deal with the frustration of having a small group of patients one week counterbalanced by a large group the next, as patient admission patterns and physical ability of patients to attend the group sessions vary. Staying tuned in to subtle changes and needs is essential in keeping these groups current and attractive.

The AIDS epidemic has created a new group of issues for the social worker to manage, such as helping patients to deal with discrimination and legal matters.

THE PHYSICAL PLANT

The Education Center is comprised of small, open counseling areas with a backdrop of audiovisual equipment, two conference rooms for group sessions, a storage area for supplies and equipment, and an area for individual work by the professional staff and support staff.

The small counseling areas are primarily used for individual interactions by one health professional with a patient and a care partner. Videocassette equipment is available in some of these counseling areas, so that videotapes can be used to supplement professional teaching.

The conference rooms are used for meetings of the various support groups, for relaxation sessions, and for those instances in which greater physical privacy is needed.

The initial design of the Education Center did not include interior walls, but instead used temporary moveable partitions to maintain an entirely open feeling. This proved to be somewhat problematic functionally, as the staff moved more and more to individual counseling sessions. Renovations then were undertaken to create the current physical setup, which provides a mix of conference room space for large groups and small individual counselling areas.

One drawback of the original design was the separation of the Therapeutic from the Education Center staff. A more fully integrated and shared staff area would have better facilitated communication and referrals between the clinical and educational professionals. Another issue that probably will need to be addressed perpetually is how to provide adequate storage space for expanding equipment and supplies.

HOURS OF OPERATION OF THE EDUCATION CENTER

Because of the importance of education to the successful operation of Cooperative Care, the Education Center is open 7 days a week, 365 days a year. Staffing patterns have shifted as a reflection of census trends. Sundays through Thursdays are usually heavier admitting days, so staffing is concentrated on those days of the week. Although the inpatient educational staff has shifted mostly to 9 A.M. to 5 P.M., the Education Center itself is still a very active place during the early evening hours. During that time period, although it is not scheduled with a heavy inpatient teaching load, the area is utilized for outpatient education classes, in topics such as preparing for childbirth.

PURCHASED OR INHOUSE MATERIALS

A frequently asked question is "Do you develop your own materials or do you purchase them from outside vendors?"

When Cooperative Care opened in 1979, there were few medication information sheets commercially produced, so Cooperative Care pharmacists developed them. Today, of course, there are a variety of commercially available drug information sheets and one needs to consider the cost of developing, updating, and reproducing them in house in contrast to purchasing them.

The Education Center staff has developed a series of information sheets on various diagnostic and therapeutic procedures to explain what a patient should expect at our facility. A specific need met by these information sheets is a description of the responsibilities faced by the care partner for a patient who is undergoing these tests or treatments during Cooperative Care hospitalization.

When Cooperative Care first opened, audiovisual materials were also purchased from outside companies. Each audiovisual educational module purchased went through a Medical Center review process to ensure that the information it contained was deemed to be correct and consistent with the policies and practices at NYU Medical Center.

If commercially available audiovisual materials meet the needs of the Education Center, considerable savings can result over starting from scratch and developing comprehensive, polished video products inhouse. Some videotapes, however, have been developed inhouse, particularly on topics that either are unique to NYU Medical Center (such as orientation films for specialized units) or on topics for which no videotapes are commercially available. The same evaluation process is used for all teaching materials, whether they are purchased outside or developed inhouse.

CONCLUSION

The philosophy underlying Cooperative Care—that patients and care partners have the right to participate fully in their care—is not mere verbiage, but a necessity for the safe operation of the unit. The Cooperative Care Education Center has the responsibility to provide the setting and the means for enabling an effective and active learning process. The outcome is directly measurable: Either the patient and care partner are able to act as a team, participating in their treatment and management during the hospitalization, or they are not. Therefore, their ability to understand and follow the therapeutic regimen at home following discharge is a known quantity, and not a blind leap of faith.

13

PATIENT SAFETY

Alan R. Schukman and Kimberly S. Glassman

CAN SAFETY BE MAINTAINED WITHOUT PROFESSIONAL OBSERVATION?

Patient safety is one of the major concerns of professionals who come to visit the Cooperative Care Unit. The question they often ask, sometimes with a strong hint of apprehension, is: "How can acute patients be safe in an environment where they are separated from the clinical staff?" The answer is that safety is assured not by involving the patient in his or her care, since an acute patient might at times be too sick to seek immediate attention when it is urgently needed, but rather by the presence and involvement of the care partner in the patient's care, supported by patient education.

PATIENT SAFETY IN TRADITIONAL UNITS

Patient safety in a traditional hospital medical or surgical nursing unit usually is maintained by the clinical staff, particularly nurses and nurse-attendants, having episodic, direct observation of the patient who is in bed in a semiprivate room. In addition to such direct observation, multiple physical tools are available to engender a safe environment. These tools consist of handrails in the hallways, side-rails on the beds, Posey vests, and call lights. Many of these devices are designed in part to restrain patients in their beds or chairs until someone is available to come to assist them.

In the Cooperative Care setting, the time spent with the patient in direct observation by a nurse is different. It is expected that the nurse not only make accurate clinical assessments, but that he or she also maintain an emphasis on education, self-care techniques, and the incorporation of the actions of the care partner into the plan of care. With patients spending most of their day independently, under the direct observation only of the care partner, a nursing assessment includes teaching basic safety needs such as wheelchair use, the use of hand rails when ambulating, rising slowly from the supine position, frequent rest periods to avoid fatigue, and knowing when to call the nurse for assistance.

VISITOR VS. PARTICIPANT

In a traditional hospital setting, the role of visitor is sometimes a setup for an adversarial relationship with the professional staff. Visitors often are put into helpless positions in unfamiliar situations, with little or no information provided for them until the overburdened staff can spare the time to discuss the visitor's concerns. If the visitors cross the unmarked boundary line into either "bothersome" or "too helpful" in acknowledging the business of the staff, they might be asked to leave. The patient is then left alone and, predictably, when the inevitable problem develops, it is perceived as a failure of the hospital staff. "If only you had let us stay . . ." says the family, implying that the patient had been neglected or maltreated, and communication and trust deteriorates.

In Cooperative Care, the role of one or many visitors is legitimized into the role of active partnership in care, not passive stranger. Care partners are welcomed into the team for many reasons. One of these is that they help the patient handle those needs that are small in the staff's eyes, but loom as large problems to the patient; for example, assistance with personal hygiene, feeding, fetching supplies, helping with nourishment, and the like. Both the patient and the care partner learn a valuable lesson: how to support each other in an acute episode, which can better prepare them to manage independently later at home. Staff gain an ally on the health care team, one who will work harder than any professional would, to ensure that their loved one is kept comfortable and safe.

The care partner is the most important source of data in evaluating patients for safety needs. The family member or friend provides the crucial link in the evaluation of the safety plan of care, as the physicians and nurses come to have faith in the reliability of the care partner's assessment of the patient's needs. All factors must be considered. Elderly couples who function independently at home often can adapt their routines to Cooperative Care. Decreased vision and ambulation are common. A wheelchair can provide as much stability as a walker. Patients with dementia can, with appropriate care partners, do remarkably well in Cooperative Care's homelike setting, where distracting stimuli can be minimized, and bonding between patient and care partner helps, combined with assistance of the nursing staff, to main optimal safety with minimal risk.

Cooperative Care has handled a wide variety of patients along with their care partners over the years, attaining a degree of safety which is considered "unusual" for even a traditional setting to achieve. It has proven to have the ability to adapt to a wide variety of needs.

THE NONAMBULATORY PATIENT

Consider the following example: An elderly couple in their nineties—a nonambulatory patient and a care partner with decreased vision—were admitted to Cooperative Care. In the Education Center, the decision was made to manage the non ambulatory patient by using a wheelchair to be pushed by the husband, despite his decreased vision. Although the patient was unable to walk long distances, her vision was fine. She was therefore able to direct her more ambulatory husband around the Cooperative Care Unit.

However, due to the advanced age of the couple, the nursing staff was concerned whether the extent of ambulation required would exceed their ability, and thus planned to have meals delivered to the room. In addition, the nurses were prepared to make room visits for assessments and treatments, whenever necessary. However, the patient and care partner refused the more "roombound" option, preferring the socialization of the patient dining room, and of the clinical areas on the 14th floor. By allowing them to keep their own routine intact, the couple's independence was well-supported in the Cooperative Care facility. A traditional unit might well have forced them into a more restricted mode of nearly bedbound immobility, with the resulting deconditioning and potential for harm.

THE VISUALLY IMPAIRED PATIENT

Most commonly, patients who are visually impaired are able to obtain a sighted care partner among their family members or friends. Sometimes, however, a blind person's sighted partner is not a human being, but a seeing-eye dog. A more detailed orientation to the facility, including a tour with a staff member, can establish a level of safety for the patient and seeing-eye dog/care partner team.

The first time a seeing-eye dog arrived in Cooperative Care there was a great deal of anxiety on the part of the professional staff. The dog was made an "auxiliary care partner," with a relative of the patient as the responsible party. After a day or two, however, the situation was so well in hand that the dog was "promoted" to rank of full care partner, although with modified meals.

THE HEARING-IMPAIRED PATIENT

Occasionally, a hearing-impaired patient has a care partner who is likewise afflicted. When this situation is faced at the time of admission to Cooperative Care, the pair are provided with special telephone equipment (TTD) for their room and for the therapeutic center, so as to ensure an effective communication link between the nursing staff, patient, and care partner. In addition, the bathroom emergency call bell is emphasized in its usefulness, as it provides an audible alert to the therapeutic center nursing station, identifying the room having trouble.

Middle-aged hearing-impaired sisters, one the patient, the other the care partner, are a recent example. The staff members quickly came to look on the use of the special telephone equipment as a learning opportunity for themselves, and enjoyed the interactions. Although in the past one of the nurse-educators was fluent in hand signing, at this time there is no full-time staff member who has this proficiency.

THE HANDICAPPED CARE PARTNER

A common scenario is that of an elderly individual entering Cooperative Care, with a somewhat confused and debilitated person tagging along behind. What is surprising is that sometimes the laggard is the care partner, and the patient is the better-appearing person. The chronically ill spouse is not currently in need of hospitalization, but how can that person be a help to the less handicapped patient? The "healthier" patient and "sicker" care partner couple often choose to be managed in Cooperative Care, as it brings peace of mind for the patient, who knows that the handicapped care partner is not being left behind, alone at home. This sense of security for the patient can really be significant.

In these instances, there is usually minimal confusion, as the homelike surrounding of Cooperative Care and the presence of the spouse is calming to both the patient and to the care partner. However, the staff comes to recognize that this couple needs more assessment and supervision by both the Education Center and the Therapeutic Center to assure that their safety needs are met. Frequent communication between the various members of the Cooperative Care staff is needed, and it also helps to ensure the shortest possible duration of hospitalization for such handicapped couples.

In order to safeguard the handicapped care partner, it sometimes is necessary to keep him or her in the core clinical or educational services area in view of the staff while the patient undergoes treatment off the unit.

HAZARDS OF THE PHYSICAL ENVIRONMENT

In the Cooperative Care setting, the environment is very much "homelike." However, the presence of complicated equipment can place the patient at risk for injury. For example, the rolling intravenous pole can narrow the corridor and impede passage. Wheelchairs can tip or roll while a transfer is being made. Even dangling wiring from a Holter monitor can introduce the patient to the potential for tripping or falling. Meticulous maintenance of all equipment is a priority. Before patients and care partners use any new equipment, they must be given thorough instruction in the Education Center, usually beginning at the time of admission. Direct observation of their initial use of such equipment is essential.

MEDICATIONS

In addition to surmounting the hazards of the physical environment, patients and care partners face the responsibility of administering medications via the Self-Administration of Medication (SAM) program. This might add worry and concern, but it unquestionably adds to patient safety. SAM overcomes the sometimes difficult task of dealing with new medications, frequent changes in dosage, or even the same medication appearing in different shapes or colors.

Patients and care partners are provided with medication teaching sheets upon admission. These sheets list the generic and trade names of the drug, the possible side effects, and common indications for use of the medication, as well as information regarding proper dosage and methods of administration. Unlike a traditional setting, patients are asked to bring all medications from home to Cooperative Care upon admission. Shortly after admission, all the patient's medications are reviewed with a pharmacist, in an individual teaching session. This not only allows the pharmacist the opportunity to assess the patient's and care partner's knowledge for self-administration, but also gives the patient the opportunity to ask many questions and to feel more at ease with the medical regimen. The nurse-clinician then provides ongoing daily assessments of the patient and care partner's ability to self-administer the medications. Changes in the medication profile are updated during the daily nursing assessments, and new medication sheets are given to the patient whenever indicated. To assist the patient throughout the stay in Cooperative Care, medication flow-sheets are given so that he/she can document which medications are taken. These serve as a compliance tool to assess the patient's handling of their current medication regime.

An important care partner function is acting as a safety net. As they have learned about the disease and its treatment along with the patient, they are equally—or more—aware of what should be done. Thus, when an error is being made, the care partner is alert to "what should be," and has been taught to question any deviation from that expectation. The bottle of medication received might contain green tablets instead of pink ones due to differences between manufacturers, but it might be the wrong drug. The care partner usually is the first to question whether this is correct. Because of the active role of the care partner with SAM, medication administration errors are nearly nonexistent.

REPORTING PROBLEMS

The Cooperative Care environment has demonstrated unequivocally that the family is very reliable in identifying and reporting problems to the professional staff. In traditional hospital units, with the exception of intensive care units, nursing observation is episodic. While the nurse is assisting one patient, the patient at the end of the hall might be beginning to fall out of bed or experiencing respiratory distress or some other major problem. In Cooperative Care, the patient is not left unattended at these times. With the care partner on the scene, routine observation is more continuous than is the case in traditional nursing units. A loved one usually is remarkably astute in identifying subtle changes in a patient's condition. Family members and close friends know the patient's "normal behavior" better than most professionals, and can spot specific changes quickly if they have been taught what to expect. Advocating for the sick family member or friend, the care partner can swiftly notify the staff in an emergency. As part of that advocacy, it might be necessary at times simply to obtain items for the patient, such as those used for comfort, that would otherwise be delayed because of their low priority for the professionals. Avoiding frustrations and delays in these "small" matters also helps to avoid the hazards of irritability and impetuous behavior which can lead to falls.

STANDARDIZATION OF PROCEDURES

Standardization of procedures is important in every unit and in every industry, but it is crucial when the patient and care partner are learning to perform a task. Variation in the technique of dressing changes, for example, can wreak havoc for a patient and care partner who have been taught one method. As learners, they feel the need for understanding a standard, and if faced with another health professional who has a different personal preference, confusion can easily ensue between what is a trivial divergence and what is an important oversight.

Thus, a common approach when meeting patient and care partner is to say "Show me how you have been taught to do this dressing," thereby accomplishing the objectives of review and maintaining continuity of training.

When confusion begins, however, the written patient education materials are handy references for the staff as well as for the patient and care partner. As "masters" of new techniques, patients and care partners become eager to demonstrate and share their knowledge and skill with the staff. The learning environment is ever-present, and a natural and nonthreatening scenario for staff and patient to learn together. The strategy is to make the patient and care partner feel "more powerful" than the staff.

EMERGENCY TELEPHONE

The standard hospital emergency procedures are followed in Cooperative Care, with a few added refinements. In most instances, the care partner alerts the nursing staff in the early stages of an emergency and, after the initial response to the room the patient is brought to the observation unit for further care. Each patient room is equipped with a telephone which is marked with frequently called hospital telephone numbers. The emergency telephone extension, "2000," is indicated in large print on each phone, and is featured prominently in Cooperative Care's patient literature. If a patient or care partner requires immediate assistance and dials extension 2000, two specially designated red telephones ring at the Therapeutic Center. Because these telephones produce a distinctive alarmlike sound, the line is always answered on the first ring. Staff then ask if this is an emergency, and the location and nature of the emergency. If it is an emergency, the clinical staff, already alerted by the different-sounding (and loud) telephone bell, are rapidly dispatched to the room with a "stat box," which contains a stethoscope, sphygmomanometer, and mask resuscitator. When the nursing staff enters the room, if more assistance is needed, a fully stocked emergency cart can be quickly delivered to the room.

If an individual has dialed extension 2000 for general information or some other non emergent reason, he or she is instructed to call back on the Therapeutic Center's general telephone extension, and the phone call is terminated. Thus, that line is reserved solely for true emergencies.

Extension 2000 has backup lines that roll over onto other telephone extensions, so a caller will not encounter a busy signal even if two emergency calls occur simultaneously.

CALL BELLS

In addition to the emergency telephone, the bathroom call bell is a totally independent second emergency call system similar to the traditional hospital call system. When a patient or care partner activates the system via the pull-cord, there is an audible and visual signal at the master station located in the Therapeutic Center. As this area is staffed at all times, a prompt response is ensured.

CARDIAC ARREST

When a cardiac arrest occurs, an advanced life support emergency team and equipment is dispatched to the site, whether it be the patient's room, the core services area or elsewhere. Full resuscitative measures are provided, including endotracheal intubation, ventilatory support, and even intra-aortic balloon pump insertion if needed. As a majority of the Cooperative Care clinical staff have had prior experience in critical care nursing, these episodes are handled more smoothly on average than on most medical/surgical units of a traditional hospital.

If circumstances permit, the patient is moved to the observation unit for emergency care, as this is more comfortable for both the patient and the staff. However, emergency treatment, including resuscitation, is provided wherever it is needed.

INFECTION PRECAUTIONS

Maintaining infection control via universal precautions under OSHA guidelines is a challenge faced by all hospitals in the present era. In the traditional hospital setting, potentially infectious patients are identified by physicians and nurses by such means as large signs on the doors and obviously placed precautionary devices which, in effect, "flag" patients as posing special hazards.

In Cooperative Care, there are no signs on patients' doors or specialized equipment in the hallway to alert personnel of any special needs. Thus, the issue of isolation on the unit must be viewed from a different angle. Respiratory isolation cannot be easily managed in an environment in which patients mingle freely with other patients and their families. Therefore, such patients are excluded from entry to Cooperative Care. In some instances, however, this information may not be available at the time of admission. With the rise of tuberculosis today, especially in metropolitan areas, this disease probably presents the greatest concern. If, during any part of the stay in Cooperative Care, a patient is suspected of having tuberculosis, he or she is immediately placed in respiratory isolation. This consists of restriction to the patient room, or the use of a demistifier tent or a mask, until transfer to the traditional part of the institution is effected. Care partners also are instructed in ways to minimize the risk of transmission, and medical evaluation is arranged for them as well.

On the other hand, isolation of patients with disorders which can be transmitted by direct personal contact, or by contaminated body fluids or stool is readily managed in the Cooperative Care setting. All patient records including the chart, escort requests, lab and radiology slips are flagged, alerting all personnel in contact with the patient. Nurse-educators provide guidelines for patients placed on any form of isolation, and teach care partners how to live and manage within those guidelines in order to minimize risk to all parties. In keeping with this level of isolation, patients are permitted to move about the entire unit without restriction, and without stigma.

24–HOUR CARE PARTNERS

Even when convinced of the feasibility of providing safe care in a Cooperative Care Unit, the skeptic says, "We could never ask patients to have a 24–hour care partner." But we do! And they come and they serve. On admission, the nurse-educator assesses the ability of the patient and care partner to manage in this environment. Our many years of experience have taught us to quickly identify who is likely to be safe, and who is not.

The patient who arrives without a care partner can be managed in a number of ways. One option is to refuse admission, which would anger the patient, the family, and the physician. Another alternative is to suggest that the patient hire a companion to act as a care partner, who is available at the times which are most essential for safety, such as in postprocedure observation. For the rare patient without any friends or family this is the most practical course of action. However, many patients arrive at the Cooperative Care admitting office stating that they have no one to act as a care partner, not having believed the information, including the printed literature, they have received, or perhaps not having had advance warning that they would be admitted, due to the urgency of their health problem. The Education Center nurse-educator and social worker help solve that problem with the patient and family. Since the care partner represents safety, and the lack of a care partner could be hazardous, this issue is addressed and solved immediately upon arrival.

CARE PARTNER NETWORKS

Although one care partner for the entire Cooperative Care hospitalization is the norm, it is not always practical in an era of economic problems and dual-career households. Therefore, a "care partner network" needs to be activated by an explanation of the purpose of a care partner and the need for assistance at various times. Family members and friends can choose shifts of time during which each individual will stay with the patient, so that others can work or plan days off around patient procedures. A network of family and friends can even take turns throughout the day and evening, thereby assisting the patient while still attending to their own lives. There are many times, for example, when the patient is undergoing a procedure or is otherwise under the care of the professionals, receiving intravenous medication or having diagnostic tests, when the presence of a care partner is not essential. As patients usually have a number of diagnostic tests in a day, when these procedures can be scheduled together, the care partner has more time to attend to other needs.

ABSENT CARE PARTNER

Ambulatory patients who live alone and have no family members nearby have the hazard of the absence of a care partner weighed in relation to the current health problems, and a continuous care partner may be deemed unnecessary. This is a collaborative decision reached by the patient, the nurse, and the physician. Ultimately, if one of these people is uncomfortable with the lack of a care partner, admission to the traditional part of the hospital may be warranted. Lacking a care partner, a patient who is scheduled to undergo an elective procedure may have the admission postponed until the care partner issue is resolved. A patient requiring urgent admission for an acute problem may be admitted directly to the Cooperative Care observation unit. Although this is the least-preferable admission option, it does allow the acutely ill patient to receive immediate treatment in Cooperative Care until a solution can be worked out.

For example, an immunosuppressed patient might call his or her physician with worrisome symptoms, then deteriorate more rapidly than expected, arriving for the admission to Cooperative Care with very advanced clinical needs. Rather than sending the patient to the Emergency Room, the observation unit is likely to be used as the hospitalization entry point. Often, the patient can be stabilized there over the subsequent 12 to 24 hours, and then be treated in the customary Cooperative Care pattern of management. Such flexibility and individual tailoring of solutions is the hallmark of the unit.

14

MANAGEMENT

Margaret L. McClure, Patricia L. Valoon, and
Theresa A. Bischoff

In many ways, managing a Cooperative Care Unit is like managing
any other health care facility. There are, however, some unique aspects
that require specific kinds of approaches and adaptations. This chapter will describe some of the different management practices that need
to be considered, along with the lessons we at NYU Medical Center
have learned and the changes we have made over time.

As with any other major program introduction, commitment and
support from the very top of the organization are essential if a new Cooperative Care Unit is to succeed. This means a great deal more than
lip service and/or approval without involvement. Clearly, how that involvement is operationalized is, to some degree, a matter of style. It
may range from management-by-walking-around to formal periodic
meetings between the executives and the management and/or staff of
the unit. There should, however, be no doubt on anyone's part that the
influential personnel of the institution are four-square behind the program and will do whatever it takes to make it thrive.

ORGANIZATIONAL STRUCTURE

Administration

Because our unit was experimental, large (104 patients) and some-what remotely located from the main part of the acute hospital, a separate administrative team was initially put into place. The hospital administrator appointed to oversee the Cooperative Care program was housed in a suite that he shared with the medical director, nursing managers, and secretary; these offices were located adjacent to the patient treatment area so that everyone was quite close to the unit's center of action.

Early on, this administrative team reported directly to the chief executive officer, who was intimately involved with the program from its inception. This relationship continued for several years and fostered confidence in this innovative approach to patient care.

Over time, Cooperative Care developed its own routines and rhythms and was no longer considered an experiment. The administrative structure evolved in such a way that the unit gradually became the responsibility of an associate hospital administrator and was eventually folded into the nursing management structure. Thus, while Cooperative Care continues to be a significant entity at the Medical Center, with one exception it currently enjoys much the same status as other patient care areas, such as the intensive care units or the obstetrical service.

That one exception is a weekly administrative team meeting. From the very beginning, when the concept of Cooperative Care began to germinate, a top-level management team met on a weekly basis to finalize the planning and later to maintain the momentum for the development and refinement of the Cooperative Care program. We so enjoyed those meetings that we have continued to hold weekly Friday lunches, which are attended by the Vice President for Hospital Operations, the Director of Nursing for NYU Medical Center, the Medical Director of Cooperative Care, and the Director of Nursing for Cooperative Care. It is during these business/pleasure lunches that many decisions are made to support the changes necessary to incorporate rapid case mix changes and new program proposals, and at times share the concepts of Cooperative Care with colleagues and friends from other institutions.

The Education Center

One subset of Cooperative Care with a particularly interesting management history is the Education Center. This area was set up as a distinct department under the direction of a nurse manager with special preparation and expertise in patient education. The staff consists of nurse-educators, social workers, nutritionists, and pharmacists.

The Education Center was designed from its inception with its own space as well as a separate professional staff. The rationale for this was based in a strong belief based on long years of nursing experience in a tertiary care center. We knew that if we hired registered nurses, and assigned them to the Therapeutic Center with responsibility for patient education, that the focus on patient education would always take a secondary position to the more demanding "hands-on care" component of nursing. We believe that this separation continues to be part of the success of the entire Cooperative Care education concept. Patients and families are more receptive to learning in this comfortable environment, which has been technically well planned, professionally staffed, and purposefully arranged to meet the needs of the learner.

Originally, the decision was made to create the department in a matrix structure; that is, the members of the various disciplines had dual reporting relationships to both the Education Center manager and the heads of their respective professional departments.

The Table of Organization of Cooperative Care shows two separate but symbiotic staffs, each reporting to administrative heads, who in turn are both responsible to the Executive Director of Nursing.

One staff is responsible for the orientation and education of the patients in the Education Center; the other, in the Therapeutic Center, for their clinical assessment and care. We will discuss each staff and explore how they relate to each other and to others within the hospital.

From the beginning, the Education Center has had a multidisciplinary staff consisting of nurse-educators, nutritionists, social workers, movement therapists, pharmacists, and recreation therapist.

Whereas the benefits for comprehensive patient care from a multidisciplinary staff have been widely praised, there are difficulties to be recognized and addressed in the administration of such a staff.

Management in the beginning was a form of matrix management. Each discipline reported to both the Supervisor of the Education Center and to their respective Director (i.e., nutritionists to Food Service; social workers to the Social Service Department; etc.). Although this appeared to be a good administrative plan, in actual practice, it did not function well. A poor working relationship developed between the Supervisor of the Education Center and some of the Directors.

To facilitate a better working relationship, the management pattern was changed in 1984, when Cooperative Care was 5 years old. The position of Manager of the Education Center was created. This position was on an administrative level with the Directors of Food Service, Social Work, and Therapeutic Recreation. The Supervisor of the Education Center reported to this position of Manager; all Education Center staff members reported to the Supervisor of the Education Center and thus to the Manager, who was charged with seeking the assistance of the appropriate Director if problems developed in professional practice. Payroll and working hours were handled by the Education Center.

Pharmacists continued to report to the Manager of the Outpatient Pharmacy, with one pharmacist rotating each day to assume the role of patient counselor in the Education Center. In this function the pharmacist was supervised by the Supervisor of the Education Center.

The then newly hired Manager of the Education Center and the other Directors were made aware of the importance of maintaining a good working relationship. They continue to work toward this end. The Supervisor of the Education Center and the Manager of the Outpatient Pharmacy became a tightly knit team, both supervising the "Pharmacist Consults" and working together on the creation of the medication sheets, the handouts for patients detailing important facts about their medications. So comprehensive was their work that the library of medication sheets numbered over 350, with the most commonly used sheets available in the traditional side of the hospital via the computer.

Reflecting the social work practice of workers who report to the Supervisor for clinical supervision, in order to continue to grow in expertise and experience in their profession, a social work supervisor was appointed by the Social Work Department. She had experience as a social worker in Cooperative Care, and met regularly with the Cooperative Care Social Workers and with the Supervisor of the Education Center. Occasionally these meetings would include the Director of Social Work and the Manager of the Education Center as well, in order to ensure good communication.

In the end, the matrix was dissolved and all the staff of the Education Center now report solely to the manager there. In order to accommodate the needs of the individual professions, a great deal of collaboration still occurs, especially in terms of hiring, staff development, and student training, but we found that greater clarity of objectives and productivity expectations were accomplished through a traditional organization structure. It probably is safe to say that regardless of structure, there must be a systematic means in place to promote appropriate input from the leadership of all the involved professions where such highly interdisciplinary staff are instituted.

Although the Education Center was initially designed as an inpatient service, one of the many benefits of a separate staff was the initiative on the part of management and staff to expand to an outpatient education service.

The program was initiated and grew because of our belief that many nonhospitalized individuals could benefit from the educational services already provided there for inpatients. This outgrowth was consistent with the philosophy of Cooperative Care that an individual has the right and, furthermore, the responsibility, to participate in his own health care. The courses offered are taught by the same staff of professionals: nurse-educators, registered dietitians, social workers, certified childbirth educators, and recreation/movement therapists. Educators supplement their teaching with written materials, audiovisual films, and other materials developed by members of the NYU Medical Center staff. When appropriate, family members also attend these courses in order to provide knowledgeable support and assistance to the patient at home. Currently, we run programs in weight management, childbirth preparation, stress reduction, smoking cessation, stretching and toning, and employee wellness forums, as well as many disease-specific educational programs.

Ancillary Services

Other areas of Cooperative Care have been traditionally structured from the outset, with work assignments accommodating the unique characteristics of the program. For example, the housekeeping staff is managed in much the usual fashion by their own supervisors; however, in Cooperative Care they assume full responsibility for all aspects of patient rooms, just as they would in a hotel setting. No member of the nursing staff takes on the ordering of linens or bed changing. These kinds of activities are wholly within the housekeeping department's domain, even on the evening and night shifts.

Food Service also has a traditional organizational structure, but a different set of responsibilities in Cooperative Care. For the most part, patients and care partners eat in a cafeteria-style dining room. Diet aides are still expected to assist with the serving of trays and removal of dirty dishes but in this case the activity occurs within one room and care partners must be serviced as well as patients. Oddly enough, this requires a somewhat different approach than in a conventional hospital unit, even though the principles are not different. For example, it is very important that the food be displayed in an attractive manner. In addition, the individual items need to be labelled as to their appropriateness for particular special diets. In this way, the educational program is reinforced and, although patients are free to select whatever they please, they do so as informed consumers.

In such an organizational environment, there is less opportunity for interdepartmental communication, chiefly because the nurses do not do as much coordination as they would in traditional inpatient settings. To overcome this, the operational supervisors from the major departments have formed a group that meets regularly to identify and solve problems together.

Medical Director

Cooperative Care has a special impact on physicians, and our unit at NYU had not been open very long before it became evident that the appointment of a director would be highly advantageous. To some extent, this was as much a marketing need as it was a clinical need.

Many members of the medical staff supported the concept of the unit early on; many more, however, had concerns as to how the system would work for their patients, especially with regard to safety issues. These worries were quite understandable and were assuaged, to a large degree, by the appointment of a highly respected attending physician who agreed to serve as Medical Director for the program.

Beyond the marketing concerns, a number of clinical/administrative issues were and continue to be greatly assisted by the presence of a committed Medical Director. These include his involvement in developing (and changing) such things as the criteria for admission, the clinical content of educational materials, and the evaluation of new programs as they arise.

In addition, the director serves as chair of a Cooperative Care Committee of the Medical Board. This committee has representatives from every service in the institution and serves as a formal review panel for policies and procedures related to clinical care. They report to the Board of Trustees through the Executive Committee of the Medical Board, and serve as an important communication vehicle as changes in practice are incorporated into the unit.

Probably everyone concerned would agree that the preponderance of changes that have occurred over time in Cooperative Care have been related to the acuity of patients who are admitted to the facility. Changing technology has facilitated our ability to care for increasingly ill patients in the homelike environment, but this requires continuous attention to the adaptation of equipment and supplies to maintain a safe, independent approach to care.

This speaks to the need for flexibility in policies and procedures, ensuring that the unit is organized in such a way as to permit and encourage evolution in keeping with patient needs.

Policies and Procedures

It may be useful to speak specifically to the kinds of policies and procedures that need to be in place for the Cooperative Care Unit. Recognizing that policies and procedures exist to regulate the environment, bringing order to potential chaos and reducing risk to the organization, it is important that these regulations not become overly rigid, especially in the early days of the unit's existence. Some risk-taking is necessary.

Two principles that should be used as guides are that regulations be user-friendly and flexible wherever they are put into place. Concerning user-friendliness, it is expected that patients will function independently with the aid of their care partners; it is then necessary to break with many long-cherished traditions. For example, a carefully conceived program must be developed for self-administration of medications, including a system for the patient to document dosages and side effects. Can a patient or care partner make a medication error? Yes. But such incidents are exceedingly rare and an error made in Cooperative Care is much more likely to be identified and corrected promptly than such an error made at home, postdischarge.

As expected, we have had to change many policies as experience has dictated. We originally had attempted some controls by mandating that patients could only be admitted to Cooperative Care as transfers from the main hospital and that all must have care partners with them 24-hours a day. It was not long before we came to realize that substantial numbers of admissions could come directly to the unit from home; and later it also became apparent that the number of hours of care partners' time needed varied from patient to patient, depending on the day's clinical activities. Subsequently, the required care partner hours were determined by the nurse after assessing the patient's condition and the plan of care. Needless to say, this has made an enormous difference in the number of family members and friends available to assist any given patient.

Another example of change over time concerned the admission of patients directly from the Emergency Room. Initially, we created a policy barring such a route, principally because we were afraid that the patients would prove to be inappropriate for the setting. Subsequently, we came to realize that many of these patients could be managed very well in the unit. Our current procedure calls for a preadmission assessment performed in the Emergency Room by the nurse manager or a senior nurse-clinician from Cooperative Care, so that everyone involved is comfortable that the environment will be suitable for the patient.

Environmental Concerns

Probably the most important feature in the Cooperative Care environment is the careful attention given to safety. Because patients and care partners are quite literally on their own, every effort is made to protect them to the extent possible.

As noted earlier, the unit is carpeted throughout and practical, yet unobtrusive, handrails are in abundance. The patient rooms actually do not appear much different from hotel accommodations, except that the bathroom is well equipped to service frail and handicapped individuals; it also has an emergency pull-cord that can be used to signal the nursing staff in the Therapeutic Center if help is needed.

Most critical is the telephone at the bedside. A separate line is dedicated purely to emergency use and the patient/care partner team is carefully oriented to it. The telephone that receives these calls in the Therapeutic Center is never left unattended. As a result, our response to serious problems, even cardiac arrests, has never proven problematic.

Other aspects of the environment are devised purely to support the notion of being user-friendly. These include the placement of refrigerators in every patient room, a laundry facility with a coin-operated washer/dryer, and soda machines.

Most unique, of course, is the unusual privacy that patients and care partners are afforded. Each room is locked and, with the exception of the maids and porters, no member of the staff enters without permission. This aspect has received very high marks from patients, particularly as they find the privacy also contributes to a quiet atmosphere that is conducive to rest and recuperation.

Staffing

Clearly, the single factor that makes Cooperative Care exceptionally cost-effective is the low staff-to-patient ratio that can be achieved because of the presence of care partners. However, although the quantity of staff may be lower than in traditional settings, it probably is safe to say that the quality must be higher.

Certain characteristics are essential for employees who work in Cooperative Care, regardless of discipline. Overall, they need to value family and loved ones and to see them as an essential part of the health care team. Although this may seem self-apparent, and is clearly a tenet preached by most professions, many individuals who work with patients view their visitors as intrusive nuisances who make demands and ask too many questions. Those who practice in Cooperative Care must be willing to give up a substantial amount of control if they are to succeed and must understand that excluding family members is simply not an option in this setting.

A second characteristic, especially important for the professionals involved, is the need for very seasoned, highly competent practitioners. To a large extent, this requirement stems from the fact that patients in Cooperative Care represent the fullest possible array of diagnoses and, therefore, require knowledgeable individuals prepared to deal with a wide variety of patient needs.

SPREADING THE PHILOSOPHY

Spreading the concepts, culture, and practices of Cooperative Care has enhanced the quality of patient care throughout the Medical Center. Our patient education tools, medication information protocols, and closed circuit television programs are utilized constantly by our professional staff for patient education throughout the institution.

One of the unique aspects of Cooperative Care that was discussed previously is the Self-Administration of Medication (SAM) program. The goal of the SAM is that the patient and/or family member will be able to articulate pertinent medication information and actually administer all of the patient's medications prior to discharge.

There are two other areas in hospitals that will adapt readily to a self-administration medication program for patients. Our experience has shown that 2 to 5% of patients in the acute rehabilitation setting are capable of demonstrating safe self-administration of medication. Another 10% of acute rehab patients, although unable to pour and administer their own medications can, using a preprinted medication sheet, go to the nurse and request the correct medication at the correct time and discuss the pertinent information about each medication. This is a modification of our original program, and is referred to by nurses and patients as self-directed medication administration.

The second area that readily adapts to a SAM program is, as you can easily imagine, the obstetrical service, where the patients are generally younger, ambulatory, and as a rule take fewer medications than most other hospitalized patients. Education related to medications utilized for pain management can be started in the prenatal classes and simply reinforced on admission.

The concept of closed circuit television has been the "dream child" of every Director of Nursing and every patient educator. In the early years, we contracted for the development of two new closed circuit television programs per year. Finding someone to participate in putting together a closed circuit television program for patient education was a real chore, because everyone was camera-shy. Now, there is a waiting list for closed circuit television programs, and staff view it as a reward when their request for proposal is approved. Currently, our programs include orientations to the main hospital, the Cooperative Care Unit, the Institute of Rehabilitation Medicine, and the Day Surgery Unit. Physicians who utilize our Day Surgery suite also use the orientation film for patients and families in their private offices. Other programs have been developed related to disease-specific or informational needs. These include "Preparing for Discharge after Open-Heart Surgery," "Understanding Diabetes," "Women's Health," "Stress Management," "Hickman Catheter Management," "Safety Shorts," "Patients' Rights," "Dispelling the Myth of AIDS," "At Risk for Heart Disease," "Understanding Hypertension," and many others.

A recent benefit to our professional staff was the inclusion of our medication information sheets on our Hospital Information System. This enables the nurse who has a patient on a specific antihypertensive drug to go into the system, pull up the medication, and print two copies of the medication information sheet to be used with the patient being discharged. The patient will receive one copy of the medical information sheet and a signed copy can become part of the patient's medical record, showing evidence that they understood the pertinent information about the drug that they would be taking when discharged.

Last, but not least, a great many of our patients are seen in the Education Center prior to admission and receive teaching related to many aspects of the care that they will be needing when they come into the hospital. For example, patients scheduled for a procedure in Day Surgery present to PreAdmission Testing. They proceed to the Education Center for teaching relating either to the type of procedure for which they are to be admitted and the aftercare related to that procedure, to diet if they are diabetic, or heart disease if they present with such a diagnosis. The Patient Education staff have created a very valuable patient service that markets the Medical Center and all our professional staff in a very positive way.

Costs

Spreading the culture, concepts and practices of Cooperative Care to other hospitals will enhance not only the quality but also the cost effectiveness of care. Health care reform places an emphasis on programs geared to health promotion, disease prevention and self-care management of chronic illness. Cooperative Care promotes all of these concepts of care at 35% less cost than a comparable number of traditional medical beds at Tisch Hospital of NYU Medical Center.

Operationally, three cost centers contribute to this reduction in operating expenses. They are 1) staffing, 2) supplies and equipment, and 3) hotel services. Staffing is 37.1% less than at Tisch, but the staffing budget is only 27% lower. This is because the professional staff is more senior, averaging 13 years of experience for nurses, and turnover in Cooperative Care has always been less than on our traditional units. For example, in 1991–1992, turnover on medical units was 16.5%, contrasted to only 9.4% in Cooperative Care. We feel that this increased knowledge and experience at the professional level is an essential ingredient for safe and cost-effective operation of a Cooperative Care venture.

The cost of supplies and equipment in Cooperative Care is nearly 48% lower than on our traditional medical units. This is primarily due to our targeted patient population, who present with a 10% lower case mix index; the construction efficiencies; and a concerted effort on the part of the staff to be cost-conscious and therefore cost-effective with supplies. The remainder of the 35% total cost reduction we enjoy is related to the hotel services (food service, cleaning, linen, laundry, and other building service componenents) in Cooperative Care.

The effect of the cost reduction in Cooperative Care on the rest of the institution is also dramatic. As managed care began to expand, NYU Medical Center found itself well positioned for that arena. We are, in fact, the lowest cost tertiary care facility and second lowest cost hospital in all of Manhattan. The cost reduction related to Cooperative Care is one of the major factors contributing to our favorable position. More programs like Cooperative Care are in order if we are to close the gap toward an integrated delivery system which decreases the fragmentation of care and reduces cost. Cooperative Care is one of our great success stories made possible, because we went beyond the walls of the traditional hospital setting and put a higher emphasis on the need to share pertinent knowledge with our consumers and their care partners to promote wellness and reduce recidivism.

15

LEGAL AND LIABILITY

Pamela Brown

The cornerstone of any risk management program is the combination of the delivery of humanistic, high-quality care with a trusting relationship by the patient and family with the professionals providing the care. Illness is characterized by social and emotional symptoms as well as by physical manifestations. The atmosphere in which care is given can affect patients and families either favorably or unfavorably. Anxious reactions to unfamiliar surroundings, with the patient and family fearing the unknown and lacking a complete understanding of what is happening or about to happen, are important components of the reaction to hospitalization. In Cooperative Care, issues related to quality of care and risk management are as obvious to the patient's family as they are to the professionals.

FAMILY AS PROTECTION

The relationship of the patient and family with professional staff frequently can have more influence over whether a liability claim is filed than does the actual course of medical treatment, its outcome, or any complications of management. Patients and families are less likely to sue those who have taken the time to establish good rapport and have expressed feelings of concern about the patient's well-being.

Family members play a key role in establishing this relationship in a Cooperative Care setting. Protection for both patients and the institution can be facilitated by effective communication between family members and the hospital staff. As active participants in the patient's care, the family members identify with the professionals as part of the care team. This can help to resolve or avoid patient complaints, improve the patient's understanding of the care provided, and identify incidents that might otherwise develop into serious grievances. The family member is more likely to articulate problems earlier than the patient would left alone in a similar circumstance. Thus, questions arise that clear the air and avoid festering frustration. In addition, the family's constant presence provides protection for the patient through continous observation of his or her care, thereby helping to prevent injuries.

Maintaining open communication, with full access to patients' medical records, helps to reduce the distrust and suspicion that could otherwise develop in some patients and their families in traditional, restrictive hospital settings. The presence of a multidisciplinary team of senior professionals, whose focus is as educational as it is curative, does much to facilitate reduction of anxiety.

THE PATIENT REPRESENTATIVE

In traditional hospital settings, when patients experience ongoing problems in dealing with frustrations relating to their hospitalization, and these problems cannot be resolved by the staff directly involved in their care, patient representatives are often contacted to communicate with the patients and their families in order to seek solutions. The purpose of the patient representative is to serve as an ombudsman for both the patients and the hospital. Their widespread success can largely be attributed to their lack of any vested interest in either party. In Cooperative Care, a very small proportion of patients, perhaps only about 5%, utilize the patient representative service. This appears to be explained by the environment of the Cooperative Care setting, which empowers patients and their families to act for themselves in seeking resolution of their problems.

RISK MANAGEMENT

Risk management is a review process which investigates incidents that occur throughout the hospital. Of the risk management indicators which are followed institution-wide, two are particularly relevant to the Cooperative Care setting in comparison to the traditional nursing units: patient falls and medication errors.

Patient Falls

Patient falls were a potential concern when Cooperative Care was first being planned, since there are no nursing personnel stationed on the patient room floors. Thus, prevention of falls is within the purview of an alert care partner, who has been given instruction in the Education Center. As the acuity level has risen over the past several years, patients are weaker and weaker, so concern over the hazard of falling in patient rooms has been continually assessed.

Table 15.1 shows the comparison of patient falls in Cooperative Care with the traditional hospital units of the Medical Center for the latest year (1991) for which complete data are available at the time of this writing. The number of falls, of course, must be judged with regard to the number of beds in each part of the institution. Cooperative Care, with 104 patient beds, has 14.3 % of the total hospital bed capacity of 726. Thus, if the risk for falling in Cooperative Care were equal to the

TABLE 15.1 Patient Falls: Year 1991

	Cooperative Care	Total Hospital	COOP/HOSP
Fall, no injury	44	609	7.2%
Minor injury	19	148	12.8%
Fractures	0	7	0.0%
Visitor injury	3	21	14.3%
Total falls	66	785	8.4%
Number of beds	104	726	14.3%
	Cooperative Care	Total Hospital	COOP/HOSP
Simple fall/bed	42.3%	83.9%	50.4%
Minor injury/bed	18.3%	20.4%	89.6%
Fractures/bed	0.0%	1.0%	0.0%
Visitor falls/bed	2.9%	2.9%	99.7%
Total falls/bed	63.5%	108.1%	58.7%

risk in traditional hospital units, it would account for 14.3% of all falls. In actuality, total falls in Cooperative Care were only 66, or 8.4% of the 785 falls in the whole hospital, or a reduction of 41.3% below that predicted. Fractures resulting from falls were nonexistent that year, contrasted with a total of seven in the traditional hospital. It is of note that visitor falls were exactly proportional in the two parts of the institution; Cooperative Care had 3 and the total hospital 21, for a 14.3% ratio precisely equal to the ratio of beds in each category. This, in effect, served as a control group, validating the experienced difference in patient falls in the two settings.

How can this difference in falls be explained? We attribute it to the presence of a dedicated care partner. It is of interest that of all falls occurring in Cooperative Care, 85% were related to toileting activities. The remaining 15% occurred while patients or their care partners were trying to reach objects, particularly their telephones, and bumped into objects such as the television or other furniture.

Medication Errors

The potential for errors in medication administration has been a concern in all hospitals. Therefore, surveillance of medication administration errors has been an ongoing part of the quality assurance program for the entire institution. Cooperative Care, with its self-administration of medication program, is particularly targeted for such review.

As seen in Table 15.2, medication errors are rare in Cooperative Care. In 1991, only 2 patients received the wrong medication, in contrast to 46 in the traditional hospital, at a ratio of 4.3%—which is 69.6% below what would be expected based on the proportion of bed capacity. Errors in dosage were present in only 3 cases, compared with 85 in the whole hospital; none had duplication of dosage, compared with 31 cases in the traditional nursing units. Total medication-related errors amounted to 9 in Cooperative Care, or 3.0% of the 299 in the institution, 79% lower than expected.

The very low incidence of medication errors in all categories is attributed to the combined efforts of the thorough educational program and the watchful involvement of patients and their care partners in the medication administration program. Thus, it is quite clear that sharing responsibility with patients and care partners adds to their safety in medication administration, rather than detracting from it. This lesson has wide applicability for enhancing the safety of medication use in hospitals throughout the country and, in our view, should be more widely emulated.

TABLE 15.2 Medication Errors: Year 1991

Category	Cooperative Care	Total Hospital	COOP/HOSP
Wrong med	2	46	4.3%
Wrong dose	3	85	3.5%
Duplication	0	31	0.0%
Omission	3	115	2.6%
Time error	1	22	4.5%
Total errors	9	299	3.0%
	Cooperative Care	Total Hospital	COOP/HOSP
Beds	104	726	
Wrong med/bed	1.9%	6.3%	30.4%
Wrong dose/bed	2.9%	11.7%	24.6%
Duplication/bed	0.0%	4.3%	0.0%
Omission/bed	2.9%	15.8%	18.2%
Time error/bed	1.0%	3.0%	31.7%
Total errors/bed	8.7%	41.2%	21.0%

Environmental Safety

Patients need to be protected from personal injury and loss of personal property. Therefore, one component of any risk management program is ensuring that an adequate security system is in place to provide a safe environment for patients and visitors. For example, the Joint Commission on Accreditation of Health Care Organizations requires that personnel entering patients' rooms have identification. In Cooperative Care, the presence of the care partner provides additional personal security in this regard.

In Cooperative Care, some transportation to diagnostic and therapeutic services, such as radiation therapy, is provided by the care partner. This requires that appropriate, clear and user-friendly directional signs be widely apparent, and that care partners receive thorough instruction in wheelchair safety. Of course, when transportation by stretcher is indicated, hospital personnel provide that service.

Quality Assurance

Accurate documentation is essential to any quality assurance and risk management program. The Medical Center has established a monitoring system whereby the completeness of medical documentation is regularly audited. For example, does the record include enough details about the patient's current status? Are the problems related to the patient's diagnosis and progress adequately addressed? Are orders written in a timely fashion? The reviews are carried out concurrently, while the patient is still in the hospital, so that problems can be corrected expeditiously.

Infection Surveillance

Infection surveillance is monitored by infection control personnel who report to the institution's Quality Assurance Committee. As described in the chapters on patient education and patient safety, prevention of infection is dealt with by a comprehensive educational program, directed at the patient/care partner team. One indication of the success of this strategy is that the rate of contamination of intravenous lines is so low in Cooperative Care that the lines are left in place an average of 2 days longer than in the Medical Center's traditional units.

CONFIDENTIALITY

Although the patient is permitted to examine his or her own medical record in Cooperative Care, looking at other people's charts is not permitted. Staff are held to the same standards of confidentiality as they are in traditional units.

In summary, the open, nonregimented setting for patients and their families provided by Cooperative Care incorporates the basic protections of a hospital into the framework of its daily operations. Patients actually are better protected and more satisfied in Cooperative Care, and this has translated into fewer legal and liability issues surfacing than is the case with traditional hospital care.

COMPLAINTS AND LEGAL ACTIONS

There is no real difference in potential liability between Cooperative Care and the traditional nursing unit. The medical and nursing staff have the same extent of accountability and responsibility for patient care in all parts of the institution. However, in Cooperative Care, the additional presence of the care partner in the patient room adds a degree of surveillance not usually present in ordinary medical/surgical nursing units. In our experience, complaints and legal actions arising in Cooperative Care have been nearly nonexistent.

Of a total of 509 complaint letters received by the Medical Center from 1985 to the present, none concerned patients from Cooperative Care. Of all the legal actions against the Medical Center during this period, none were directly related to Cooperative Care.

16

CROSS-CULTURAL AND SOCIOLOGICAL PERSPECTIVES

Esther Chachkes

A patient enters a hospital not only with a bodily malfunction or illness, but with a particular set of beliefs and values about illness and
treatment based on a sociocultural affiliation; and people of diverse
cultural and ethnic backgrounds become patients. In some ethnic
groups, these beliefs and values differ significantly from those of
mainstream American scientifically based medical practice. Medical
bureaucracies, including hospitals, reflect American cultural perspectives concerning the cause and meaning of illness, effective treatment,
and the organization of care, as well as expectations regarding appropriate patient and health professional behavior (Barker, 1992; Good &
Good, 1981; Lewis, 1981; Mechanic, 1968). Patients may expect health
care professionals to react in ways that are culturally familiar to
them, just as health care professionals can be confused about patient
reactions that appear at odds with their own cultural values and the
hospital's methods. It is assumed, therefore, that increased knowledge

of and sensitivity to sociocultural factors will contribute to a more effective and relevant approach to medical care, and will enhance the patient–professional relationship.

CULTURAL VALUES AND BELIEFS

Cultural values provide the framework for rules that govern patient roles, the nature of help-seeking behavior, preferences regarding interactional styles, communication patterns between patients and health care professionals, and the degree and nature of family involvement. Cultural values also dictate how the patient and the family will react emotionally to the illness and with what level of intensity (Harwood, 1981).

In all cultures, there are particular models to explain the cause of disease. Mainstream American views generally credit biological and physical reasons for the onset of disease, but in other cultures, disease may be viewed fatalistically as "God's punishment" or as supernaturally induced. Disease may be thought of as stress-related; and its onset influenced by tension, worry, or poor interpersonal relationships. In some cultures disease is interpreted as a product of imbalances of bodily states or environmental conditions, or as a result of certain unacceptable social behaviors (Congress & Lyons, 1992; Good and Good, 1981; Harwood, 1981; Low, 1984).

Similarly, there are culturally determined notions about methods for the alleviation of illness, frequently based upon culturally influenced notions of bodily functions. The Latino "hot-cold" theory of folk medicine and Chinese notions about drafts and winds are two examples. Spiritualistic rituals, herbal therapies, medicinal potions, and a variety of folk medicine interventions exist in many cultures (Harwood, 1981).

Cultural values also determine the way in which symptoms are acknowledged and interpreted. Culturally appropriate expressions of symptoms vary as do experiences of pain: an emotional expression of pain is acceptable in many cultures, but would be frowned upon by ethnic groups where a more stoic response is the cultural norm. In addition, expressions of psychological stress and mental disturbances are permitted in some cultures but not in others. In Chinese culture, for example, because mental illness is stigmatized, psychic pain is more frequently somaticized (Congress & Lyons, 1992). The experience of "nerves," commonly seen in many cultures, can be symptoms related to anger, family breakdown, or social isolation, depending upon the cultural group (Barker, 1992; Good and Good, 1981; Harwood, 1981; Low, 1984).

FAMILY ROLES

Of particular significance are cultural norms that define family roles and the family's involvment in the health status of individual patients. The family is critical in influencing the course and outcome of illness and is an integral part of the patient's experience (Barker, 1992).

The family historically is an individual's primary social unit, providing a network for protection and support. Few social institutions are as significant as the family . The psychosocial consequences of illness and the role of the family in facilitating coping and adaptation at every stage of the illness is well documented (Caroff & Mailick, 1985). The family plays a critical role in the patient's ability to manage the illness, including the hospitalization, the predicted course of the illness, and the continuity of care that will be required after hospitalization.

Illness often has a profound impact on family life; roles may change, and the nature of the relationships within the family and the quality of those relationships may be seriously altered. A family's ability to cope with illness is influenced by the degree of social and community support available to it. It is assumed that families do better when more support is available. Small nuclear families, families isolated from extended kinship systems, and one-adult or single-parent families are probably at higher risk than those that are surrounded by the nurturing care of an extended group.

The psychosocial stress experienced by the family also will be influenced by the nature of the diagnosis, the severity of the illness, and the caretaking needs of the patient. Other factors contribute to the situation as well: the age of the patient; the point at which the illness occurs in the life cycle of the patient and of the family, and the intrafamilial transactional patterns that mark how families communicate with each other, manage conflict, and tolerate emotional reactions.

Family systems are complicated, for they may encompass nonrelatives who traditionally are expected to provide parental or caregiving functions. Godparents are one example, as are domestic life partners in both homosexual and heterosexual relationships and others who play significant roles in a patient's life.

Families also vary in the degree to which they are able to provide support, ranging from close, supportive systems to alienated and isolated ones. Most families, however, are able to provide some line of defense against the stress of illness and hospitalization. Despite a range of functional capacities, the majority of families mobilize to provide both emotional and concrete assistance to the patient and to each other. However, not all families are able to sustain an ill family member. Families who have been chronically dysfunctional may be unable to manage the increased stress.

To work successfully in the patient's interest, health care providers must enlist the strength of the family system and integrate families into the plan of care of the patient; this requires allowing their participation in the daily hospital routine of patient care.

In discussing the impact of culture, however, it is important to recognize that cultural patterns represent broad generalities. On the individual level, there is a wide variation, and notions about illness and patient care are subjective and personal as well as culturally bound. An individual may fit a typical pattern or may deviate widely from expected cultural behaviors. Differences in education, life experiences, temperament, and socioeconomic class all influence the way in which an individual will adhere to cultural norms. Therefore, not all members of specific cultural and ethnic groups respond in the same way (Chachkes & Jennings, in press).

Furthermore, the degree of acculturation is an important component in the variance in a patient's accommodation to American values and, therefore, to the American biomedically based system of health care. For ethnic minorities, the situation is even more complicated by issues of language, discrimination, social class, minority status, or refugee or immigrant status, and past experiences with war, political repression, nutritional deprivation, and persecution (Chau, 1991; Ho, 1991).

COOPERATIVE CARE

The New York University Cooperative Care Unit is uniquely suited to provide an atmosphere in which cultural differences are recognized and accepted. In the Cooperative Care model, the family as care partner is an integral aspect of the delivery of care from admission. The family is there to provide emotional support and to learn, from the beginning, essential aspects of managing the illness. Also, because patient and family education is central to carrying out the philosophy of Cooperative Care, misconceptions, myths, and false information can be reversed. Furthermore, the strong emphasis on education and self-management allows nurses, doctors, and other health care professionals to assess more fully the degree of adherence to cultural beliefs and to take into consideration the patient's conceptual models of disease and treatment (Harwood, 1981). Cultural values and attitudes can then be incorporated as necessary to facilitate medical compliance and to minimize the risk of poor self-management once a patient is discharged. Enhanced educational interventions also allow health care professionals to work more successfully within these culturally based systems.

In addition, the Cooperative Care model supports a psychosocial approach, so that other factors, such as language issues and social conditions, which contribute to understanding treatment protocols and to learning self-management are more readily identified. The result is a more ethnically sensitive approach to health care.

SOCIOCULTURAL THEMES AND PATIENT CARE

The Latino Patient and Family

In discussing the social customs of Latinos, it is important to note that although most Latino groups share common cultural values and norms, there are differences between the various groups based on country of origin and social history. The terms "Hispanic" or "Latino" have been used to refer to all people from countries with historic ties to Spain. Latinos, though, have a strong sense of community; country of origin and national identity are important aspects of self-identification and pride. National differences do exist in diet, ways of life, political conditions, socioeconomic conditions, climate, and many other distinguishing factors ("Hispanic Health: Time for data, time for action," 1991).

Latinos also are of varying skin color, and not all Latinos speak Spanish. Some Latinos are bilingual, but many second-generation Latinos do not speak Spanish well while others speak no Spanish at all. Despite these differences, however, there are key cultural patterns that are shared.

In most Latino communities, the family is the center of social support. Family ties are to an extended kinship system that includes distant relatives, godparents, and close friends. Although there are some differences in Latino groups in the autonomy of the nuclear family, maintaining close relationships with the extended family is expected and highly valued.

In Mexican families, for example, closeness between parents and children is particularly strong and less support is expected from the greater kinship system. In other Latino groups, the extended family is a significant source of security and support. However, all Latino families rely upon each other for emotional nurturance, and there is a strong sense of obligation to help each other. The Latino family, therefore, considers the needs of the individual family member, including health problems, to be a family affair. It is not uncommon for individuals to consult with other family members before important health care decisions are made.

Important decisions about seeking medical help, hospitalization, and long-term care are made by the family group. Diagnosis and treatment recommendations will be discussed with the entire family before they are followed. It is expected that family members will accompany the patient to the hospital and to doctors' appointments. Medicine may be shared with friends or relatives, particularly if a prescription is found to have been helpful (Culturlinc Corporation, 1991). Health care providers must remember that in communicating with a patient, the communication is indirectly with the family as well.

Intimate matters are discussed within the family, but less frequently with individuals outside the family system. Issues that cause guilt or shame are not easily shared, and strong emotional reactions may be expressed without revealing the real source of distress (Dillard, 1983).

Gender differences also influence health care behavior. Latino cultures typically are based on concepts of "machismo" that emphasize the superior position of men in the social order. A double standard of sexual behavior and differences in power in relationship to sexual behavior are characteristic gender differences. This is particularly significant in the treatment of AIDS, as women often are unable to influence safer sexual practices. However, the concept of machismo does incorporate the responsibility of the man to protect his family and to provide adequately for them, and recent health prevention messages have been targeted to Latino men on this basis.

For the Latina woman, "Marianism" or "Marylike" behavior is a central theme. The good woman places motherhood as central in her life and devotes herself to her children. Motherhood is venerated in Latino culture, and children are very important to both women and men. The consequences of this are often seen in pediatric wards, where the involvement of mothers in the care of their children is critical. This involvement also can extend to adult children who are ill (Guendelman, 1990).

Latino cultural attitudes toward interpersonal relationships, and especially toward authority figures, highly influence interactions with health care providers. *Simpatico* is a value that relates to the importance of politeness, respect, and diplomacy in personal relationships.

Direct confrontation and criticism are considered inappropriate behaviors. Latinos frequently will appear to agree with someone, despite holding a different opinion, in order to offer a *simpatia* response. Similarly, *respeto*, the respect given to authority figures, can lead to a deferential approach to those persons who represent authority, such as doctors. Although one must be respectful and polite, appearing deferential does not mean that the physician's advice will be followed.

Religiosity is an important aspect of Latino life. After the family it provides the greatest source of emotional support. Most Latinos are Catholic, although there are a significant number of Protestants, often from fundamentalist sects such as Pentecostal, Seventh Day Adventist, and Jehovah's Witnesses. The norms of Catholic behavior, however, including attitudes toward sexual behavior, sex education, birth control, and homosexuality are powerful influences in Latino life. Religion also influences fatalistic attitudes. Many Latinos view illness as "God's will" brought on by previous or current sinful behavior, or as a result of suffering that is intrinsic to the human condition. One of the most common responses to illness is its attribution to divine punishment. This fatalistic acceptance of illness and of death can be interpreted as a giving in to fate. This contradicts the value most often held by the American medical profession which is to "fight" the illness; and not "surrender" to it. Tensions can escalate when physicians want to work more energetically toward the alleviation of the condition while the patient and family assume an attitude of acceptance of the condition (Guendelman, 1990; Kalish & Reynolds, 1976).

Latinos tend to view health holistically, as a result of the interaction of emotional, physical, and interpersonal factors. An upset in one aspect, such as a strong emotional experience, can create a physical illness. Maintaining the balance is critical. Conversely, physical ailments can be described in cultural terms that appear to suggest an emotional base. For example, the *atague* or hysterical outburst is an accepted way to express strong emotions, fear, and anxiety. Latinos also may complain of *susto* or fright sickness. However, these complaints also can be ways of describing physical symptoms (Harwood, 1981).

The "hot–cold" theory of good health (not related to actual temperature) in which there is a "balance between the body humors" is a well-known Latino health belief system. Blood and bile are "hot," whereas phlegm and black bile are "cold." Food and medicines are labeled as "hot" or "cold" and a proper maintenance of temperature is important in healing (Culturelinc Corporation, 1991; Delgado & Humm-Delgado, 1982). It is important, in respecting this cultural view, to prescribe medicines that do not appear to conflict with the theory.

Many Latinos seek alternative supports to Western medicine, particularly if the patient does not appear to be responding to medical treatment. Folk healers play an important role in alleviating stress. There are several types of folk healers, including the spiritualist, *santero*, herbalist, *santeguador*, and *curandero*. Although there are some minor differences in the practices and beliefs of these folk healers, all address several aspects of distress, including the interpersonal, emotional, and physical. All assist the individual in alleviating anxiety and provide protection and guidance.

The spiritualist is viewed as someone who can manage supernatural elements, which may be the cause of distress, and offset their influence on an individual. The *santero* diagnoses presenting physical ailments and uses life readings as a diagnostic tool. The *santero* may use herbs, candles, or dietary advice, and prescribe home remedies. The herbalist will prescribe herbs for medicinal purposes in order to maintain an equilibrium of "body humors." The *botanica* where herbs and candles are sold is a visible presence in the barrios throughout the country. The *santiguador* specializes in intestinal ailments and various body aches, and the *curandero* promotes the individual's connection to God and culture (Delgado & Humm-Delgado, 1982; Rivera, 1990).

Common to all these healers is a belief in spiritualism and in a spirit world that includes both good and bad spirits who can influence how people will behave (Delgado & Humm-Delgado, 1982). *Espiritismo*, or spiritualism, is an amalgam of Catholicism and native beliefs (with roots in the West African Yoruba religion) originating over 500 years ago at the time of the Spanish conquest (Rivera, 1992). Spiritualism incorporates a holistic view that involves aspects of body, spirit, and mind. It is important for doctors to recognize the significance of spiritualistic beliefs and practices and to accept these as legitimate cultural preferences.

In summary, health care institutions must strengthen the ability of Latino families to participate in the care of the patient, to be a partner in health care decisions, and to be present in the health care environment. Bilingual information that also is culturally relevant must be provided and, whenever possible, Spanish-speaking health care providers should be available. Sensitivity to attitudes about illness and culturally determined health beliefs, the use of folk healers, and culturally linked communication patterns will enhance the doctor–patient relationship and foster trust, increasing the likelihood of medical compliance.

Soviet Jewish Emigres

Jewish emigres from the former Soviet Union are a recent immigrant group, having arrived in greater numbers during the last 15 years. Their immigration was voluntary, but motivated mainly by issues of political fear and anti-Semitism.

Notions about economic betterment in America also were influential in the decision to emigrate. After the decision was made, most Russians experienced more and more exclusion from Soviet society, including economic losses.

For these immigrants, many emotional stresses and difficulties accompanied the immigration experience. Their losses included friendships, the protection of the extended family, and the security of an economic system with guaranteed employment and free education and medical care. In addition, many immigrants arrived in the United States with unreal expectations of the social and economic system of this country and were unprepared for the emphasis on individualistic and competitive values, dependency and compliance having been promoted as virtues under the Soviet system (Brod & Roberts-Heurtin, 1992; Hulevat, 1981).

These cultural themes of dependency and compliance permeate family life as well. Russian infants, although nurtured and given a great deal of physical contact, also are swaddled and constricted, and childrearing practices tend to foster enmeshment. Autonomy appears to be ambivalently encouraged (Belozersky, 1990; Hulevat, 1981), and conflict surrounds independence.

As a result, Russian families tend to be close and tightly knit. This tendency also was fostered by certain aspects of Soviet life, including housing shortages which kept adult children and their spouses and children living with parents. Furthermore, as a way of surviving under an authoritarian government, where those who can be trusted are few, families became quite dependent upon each other for financial, emotional and social support. In the Soviet Union, for example, connectedness was reflected in the expectation that children would take care of their elderly parents. Few nursing homes exist, and many elderly Russians have emigrated with their children (Brod & Roberts-Heurtin, 1992).

Immigration can have a powerful impact on family structure which often is greatly altered. Children learn English more rapidly and are integrated into the new culture more quickly. Parents tend to depend more on children under these circumstances, and role reversal is com-

mon. This is exacerbated when the parent is unable to find suitable
employment that matches the status he or she had in the Soviet Union
(Belozersky, 1990).

Attitudes toward authority also derive from life under the Soviet regime. Although it is not always expected that authority figures will be
nurturing and supportive, Russians tend to be less trustful and less
optimistic about those in authority than do Americans. As a result, interactions with authority figures are ambivalent. It is expected that
authority can be manipulated, bribed or pressured—demanding and
manipulative behavior is an adaptive way of getting one's needs met.
And, if it is considered too dangerous to interact with authorities, the
strategy is to ignore or avoid them (Brod and Roberts-Heurtin, 1992;
Wheat, Brownstein, & Kvitash, 1983).

Government agencies and voluntary organizations, including hospitals, also represent authority situations. Doctors in particular are im-
bued with omnipotence and authority. Doctor–patient relationships
are frequently characterized by issues of distrust and ambivalence.
The offer of help is greeted with skepticism, and developing a helping
relationship can be a real challenge.

Many health care providers describe Russian patients as "demanding and complaining." These behaviors, though, are often the result of
having coped with the Soviet system of care as well as cultural expressions of dealing with illness and surviving the system. Doctors have
learned that conflicts can arise in timing and scheduling, patient–
practitioner relationships, signing medical release forms or other papers, medication, and compliance as well as preferences for inpatient
care. (Wheat et al., 1983). For example, when appointments are missed
and patients are asked to reschedule, they may feign illness in order to
be seen immediately. This pattern developed because in the Soviet Union, clinics are open for set hours. If patients are not seen on that day
the clinic closes nonetheless. As a result, there are long waits for appointments and, frequently, scheduled appointments are not honored.
Under these conditions, many patients have learned to come late and,
if necessary, to present with a sense of urgency in order to be seen.

Physician relationships are based on the authoritarian model of the
Soviet Union. Diagnoses often are not discussed, and patients do not
understand what treatments have been administered and why. Cancer, in particular, is never openly talked about. Soviet doctors do not
share information about prognosis. Patients, therefore, consider it improper to question a physician, and physicians who offer varying approaches to treatment may be viewed as incompetent.

Furthermore, signing consent forms is a new procedure. Medical
consent is not required in the Soviet Union as choice in treatment is

not fostered (Oltarsh, 1991). The request to sign a form that is not easily understood, is unfamiliar as a procedure, and is a requirement of an authority about whom one has ambivalent feelings, may very well be met with distrust.

Medical tests and diagnostic procedures are not easily available in the Soviet Union and are generally reserved for the very ill. As a result, arrangements for tests and procedures may be met with anxiety and must be carefully explained. Medicine, as well, often is rationed and frequently not used for minor symptoms. It tends to be taken symptomatically and passed around to friends. Such outdated medical procedures as cupping (the application of hot glasses to increase circulation via a vacuum), folk medicines, including herbal remedies such as valerian, and mustard plasters are still in use. Although most of the system of health care is primitive compared with the American system, with shortages of supplies and poorly trained health care personnel, the highest level of medical care is available for high-ranking officials (Holden, 1981).

Russian health beliefs tend to view the cause of illness as a result of social and environmental factors. Russians often cite their own experiences with war, immigration, and problematic political systems as the basis for their illness. This view emphasizes the psychosocial aspects of health care (Brod & Roberts-Heurtin, 1992).

Illness also is considered very serious, and any levity or joking is seen as a sign of lack of respect and an indication that the illness is not being handled responsibly. Furthermore, smiling is reserved as a form of communication between close friends and relatives. It is not expected behavior between patient and health care provider. Attempts on the part of nurses to comb patients' hair or to start lighthearted conversations are misunderstood and patients often react as if they have been insulted (Wheat et al., 1993).

Notions of appropriate professional behavior also extend to dress and age. Young housestaff may be greeted with distrust as wisdom and experience are more valued than youth and current knowledge. Informality of dress also is suspect. Proper professionals in the Soviet Union wear uniforms. The uniform serves to underscore the formal and authoritarian nature of the physician role. In addition, physicians in the Soviet Union are employees of the State, and as such they are viewed as government officials who are expected to be in charge and to act in a paternalistic manner. Patients do not expect to be included in decisions regarding tests, operations, medications, and other diagnostic or treatment decisions. They may interpret such inclusion as a sign that the doctor does not understand what he or she is doing. The use of specialists is one way Russian patients deal with their distrust of young housestaff or their concerns with the adequacy of American care (Bord & Roberts-Heurtin, 1992; Wheat et al., 1983).

In the Soviet Union, medical care is organized quite differently from ours. Primary care frequently is delivered by a physician assistant and generally is very basic and often inadequate. The next level is outpatient care at a clinic, which may be far from home and is not considered to be of high quality. Hospital care usually is given at a nonteaching hospital, with academic hospitals offering care primarily to interesting cases. Only the highest officials receive a level of care that is comparable to the American medical system. This organization of care influences the Russian immigrant's view of the American system. Hospital stays in the Soviet Union are longer than in this country, where the push for faster discharges—a product of the current American prospective payment system—is viewed as poor quality care. Because Russian health care providers are so poorly paid, bribery or tips for services is not uncommon. Russians have difficulty believing that American care will be rendered at the highest level without a gift or tip (Wheat, et al., 1983).

For many Russian emigres, self-management of illness is not considered important. Their experience with the Soviet system of medicine, combined with a general tendency to dismiss personal responsibility for care, complicates their ability to learn the skills of self-management (Bord & Roberts-Heurtin, 1992). The challenge in providing care to Russian immigrants is to be able to create a trusting relationship, minimize dependency, and involve the patient and family more in the decisionmaking processes related to treatment and care. In order to do this, it is critical to understand the degree of loss and sense of inadequacy that immigration has imposed. In addition, substantial differences in the delivery of health care and in the nature of doctor–patient relationships dictate a thorough orientation to and explanation of the American health care system and of expectations related to medical compliance, keeping of appointments, and valued patient-provider cooperation.

Chinese-American

The Chinese-American community is a diverse one composed of groups who immigrated to this country from different parts of China, as well as Taiwan, Hong Kong, and various other Southeast Asian communities. A number of different languages are spoken, including Cantonese and Mandarin, and immigrants have come from rural as well as urban areas. Differences in geography, language, and socioeconomic experience contribute to the variety of ethnic traditions that characterize the community. However, there are many cultural similarities and many shared cultural values.

A number of traditional values have been cited as typical of all Chinese-American groups. These include: attitudes toward authority, particularly within the family, in which devotion, loyalty, respect, and deference are central components; the importance of self-restraint and self-control, which minimize the opportunities for disrupting the family's harmony with strong emotional expressions; and the discouragement of individualism in favor of the interests of the family group or social group, placing individual needs secondary to those of the family (Dillard, 1983).

Chinese culture is family-centered, and the Chinese family promotes strong kinship bonds. Family relationships are based on Confucian principles that stress specific roles and proper relationships with established responsibilities and obligations (Shon & Ja, 1982). The family is patriarchal in structure and fathers exercise the main authority. Parents expect to be respected.

Considerable emphasis also is placed on maintaining family honor. An individual who behaves in a manner that reflects poorly on the family's character shows disrespect. Individuals who perform poorly in school, are socially disruptive, or exhibit signs of mental illness bring shame upon the family (Dillard, 1983; Muller & Desmond, 1992). Because the family is viewed as a continuum of relationships, shame reflects on preceding generations as well as on future ones. This value is so powerful that shaming of the individual is often used to reinforce the prohibition against disrespectful or undesirable behavior (Kwan-Lorenzo & Ader, 1984; Shon & Ja, 1982).

Gender differences are pronounced in Chinese culture. Sons are valued more than daughters. Women generally hold a subordinate position and are expected to be obedient, unselfish, and timid (Kwan-Lorenzo and Adler, 1984; Mo, 1992). Women are expected to honor and obey their fathers, then their husbands, and finally their sons (Shon & Ja, 1982). In the traditional Chinese family, unmarried women are considered outsiders, because they will leave when they marry to join the household of their husband. For women who remain unmarried, there is no acceptable social place within the family (Mo, 1992).

Women also are expected to be modest, and this attitude can create barriers when medical examinations are conducted by male doctors. It is very important to understand this emphasis on modesty and to approach female patients accordingly, explaining fully what will be done and for what purpose (Harwood, 1981).

Gender differences also incorporate the concept of male strength and female weakness. This is an ancient one in Chinese culture, based on the belief of yin and yang, opposing aspects of the universe. Yang is considered the embodiment of goodness, strength, and superiority (male) and yin as the embodiment of weakness (female). Men, therefore, are considered stronger and superior and women, weaker and inferior (Harwood, 1981; Mo, 1992).

Chinese traditional medicine also adheres to the yin-yang concept stressing harmony and balance; illness is viewed as a disruption of this equilibrium. Balance can be disrupted by internal forces related to temperament, emotions, or age or by external influences such as social stresses or weather conditions. Other ideas relate to beliefs about "wind" (which can enter the body harmfully), "hot/cold systems" (the proper balancing of "hot" and "cold" elements such as foods, emotional states, and temperatures) "poison" (irritating substances), "blood and Ch'i" (blood and Ch'i, or "life force," must flow smoothly through the body) and "fright" (a childhood illness) (Harwood, 1981; Mo, 1991; Muller & Desmond, 1992). Many of these concepts are not so alien to those of Western medicine, and allow Western treatments to be accepted. For example, because "wind" can cause illness, airborne pollen is easily accepted as an explanation for allergies (Harwood, 1981). With these traditional concepts in mind, it is important to understand the reaction of Chinese-American patients to room air conditioners or other "wind"-producing machinery, food and drink, and even the recommendation to bathe or wash one's hair (Harwood, 1981).

Other cultural values influence the interaction between patient and professional. Harmonious interpersonal relationships dictate a more indirect style of communication, as directness could lead to disagreement and therefore to disrespect. This cultural value is at variance with American attitudes, which stress frank and direct discussion. Furthermore, Chinese tend not to express strong emotions publicly, and consider it appropriate to bear suffering and stress quietly (Lee, 1982; Shon & Ja, 1982).

In addition, these differences in communication styles are significant in situations when truth-telling and discussions of death are critical. For example, contemporary American medical ethics now support truth-telling, and American physicians believe that individual patients have a right to know about their illness and to make decisions regarding their own care. In Chinese culture, however, patients are considered vulnerable and must be protected; mention of death might incur "bad luck" and signify the end of hope (Lee, 1982). To tell someone that he or she is seriously ill or dying, then, may be dangerous. This belief can create difficulties in discussing DNR orders with the individual patient, or in implementing the Health Care Proxy legislation, where issues related to the termination of treatment are openly introduced.

Also, it is the family who expects to be informed about the patient's condition, and they may not believe it is in the patient's best interests to know about the condition (Muller & Desmond, 1992). Harwood (1981) suggests that the doctor solicit the family's permission to tell the patient, or speak with the patient alone so that the patient can still act as if the diagnosis is not known when in the presence of the family.

Problem-solving patterns identify the family as the primary social unit. It is the family that is considered the appropriate source for all the health care decisions of individual members. The autonomy of the individual is not a cultural norm. The family fully expects to be involved in determining the choice of professional and treatment and to make the decisions related to the withdrawal of heroic treatment interventions (Muller & Desmond, 1992).

The Chinese also have a strong system of traditional medicine that includes treatment of illness through such interventions as acupuncture, exercises, herbal medicines, diet, and remedial massage. However, many Chinese are able to utilize both Western medicine and Chinese medicine, and cultural beliefs can often incorporate medical practice based upon Western biological concepts.

In summary, health care professionals who approach Chinese families with an understanding of the importance of hierarchical relationships will be better able to forge a trusting relationship. Respect for family roles with inclusion of appropriate family members, sensitivity to communication, and decision making patterns, and knowledge of health care beliefs are critical in maintaining proper patient-professional interactions.

These ethnic groups are offered as paradigms of how cultural values and ideas can influence behavior related to illness and treatment. It is not possible to provide health care successfully within the American medical system without understanding variances in beliefs and norms. Health care professionals must find a way to incorporate family members into the health care system and to provide culturally sensitive and relevant educational interventions.

SUMMARY

The preceding ethnographic descriptions of Latino, Russian emigrant and Chinese-American families are offered as illustrations of the interplay of sociocultural themes with patient care, particularly those cultural norms related to family life and health care beliefs.

In cultures such as Latino, Chinese, and Russian, where the family's presence is critical to the patient's sense of well-being, Cooperative Care is without doubt of immeasurable value, because it approaches hospitalization as an extension of the patient's care at home (Grieco et al., 1990). Education, teaching, and support all foster a positive attitude toward the hospitalization and minimize feelings of mistrust. The system is more flexible, more personal, and more humane. The experience, therefore, promotes the unity of the family and encourages a network of support.

17

EVALUATION

Joyce Mamon, David M. Levine, and
A. Judith Chwalow

A plan to evaluate Cooperative Care as an innovation in the delivery of health care was built into the plans from the outset of the program (Chwalow et al., 1990). The data and results derived from the evaluation were expected to capture the process and outcome of the intervention. Process measures were used to determine whether modifications or redefinition of the program were necessary. Outcome measures were used to judge its effectiveness. In order to examine these two aspects well, it was considered essential that members of the Cooperative Care staff and the evaluators together identify the key evaluation measures to be used in the study. In order to avoid any bias by the professionals who were involved in the day-to-day operation of the program, the evaluation was conducted solely by an independent group. Evaluation of such an innovation was considered vital in helping to determine what changes would be needed to further improve Cooperative Care as a health care delivery system.

The approach to the study was developed jointly by a team from the Johns Hopkins University School of Hygiene and Public Health and the leadership of the New York University Cooperative Care Center. The primary hypothesis to be tested was whether a Cooperative Care program emphasizing patient education, patient participation in care, and support from a care partner was a cost-effective alternative to the traditional hospital's staff-intensive form of care. The evaluation design utilized a clinical trial approach, in which patients and care partners were randomly assigned to either Cooperative Care or traditional care at the Tisch Hospital of NYU Medical Center. The major variables investigated were consistent with the objectives of the Cooperative Care program in regard to enhancing patient understanding, satisfaction, and adherence to treatment, while providing less costly care, without any increase in subsequent rehospitalization or decline in health or functional status. Virtually all patients approached agreed to participate.

Sources of data included a screening interview, telephone interviews 1 and 6 months after discharge, and mailed patient surveys 9 and 12 months following discharge. Approximately 300 individuals were assigned to each group. Both groups were comparable in sociodemographic and clinical characteristics. More than 75% of the patients in the study were males. The average age was 59, and the mean educational level was 13.7 years. In terms of clinical characteristics, the largest number of patients were admitted for cardiovascular disease. Other primary diagnoses included cancer, chronic pulmonary disease, and chronic gastrointestinal disease such as peptic ulcer, colitis, or diverticulitis. The experimental and control groups were comparable with regard to reason for hospitalization, the number of symptoms upon admission, their functional status, dietary restrictions, smoking habits, and the number of medications taken at the time of discharge. Because Cooperative Care was less staff-intense, there was a concern that physicians would selectively transfer only healthier patients, which might bias the analyses. The data indicated that this did not occur, but that the patients transferred to Cooperative Care appeared by clinical measures to have been sicker than matched patients remaining in traditional hospital units and not transferred.

The process evaluation indicated that the Cooperative Care program was successfully implemented and well accepted by care partners, patients, and their physicians. Patients and care partners participated in designated educational activities more than 95% of the time. A significantly higher proportion of experimental (i.e., Cooperative Care) patients, as compared to the control (traditional hospital care) patients, reported having received dietary information. Likewise, Cooperative Care patients reported having had more contacts and more sources regarding medications, and were given more types of information about the frequency, use, and possible side effects of those medications. In addition, Cooperative Care patients reported having had more sources regarding information about their disease process and the care required for managing the illness. This was associated with an increased understanding by patients and care partners of their illness and treatment.

Cooperative Care patients found the information provided to be significantly more useful than did the control patients. The experimental (Cooperative Care) care partners also indicated, to a significantly greater extent than the control care partners, that the information provided was very useful in the management of the patient's health (p < 0.001). The experimental care partners also were significantly more knowledgeable than were control care partners about the kinds of medication the patients were taking, their indications for use, how the medication worked, and what should be done if medications were missed (p < 0.001). Patients in Cooperative Care were more knowledgeable about such areas as diet, physical activity, and medication-taking, compared to the control group. In keeping with this increased understanding, more than 95% of patients and care partners were involved in taking increasing responsibility for managing their diet, physical activity and medication-taking. This was important in preparing patients to meet their responsibilities at home following discharge.

Patients in Cooperative Care also were more likely to discontinue smoking and to adhere to dietary recommendations. These effects were particularly notable with sicker patients, and with less well-educated individuals. Although at 1 month after discharge both the experimental and control groups had high success rates on smoking cessation, a full 85% of Cooperative Care patients were still not smoking 6 months following discharge, compared to only 66% of the traditional hospital patients.

With regard to outcomes, no significant differences between groups were seen in functional status, as measured by the Activities of Daily Living Scale (ADL), Instrumental Activities of Daily Living (IADL), Mobility (MOB), and Social/Communication Activities (SOC), with the majority of patients being fully functional at 1, 9 and 12 months after hospitalization. At the same intervals, there were also no significant differences in terms of bedbound or restricted activity days, or not being able to work. About 95% of all patients had returned to work within 6 months. Analysis indicated no significant differences in the percentage of patients who were re-hospitalized, in their utilization of emergency rooms, home care or ambulatory care services, or in the development of new health conditions. Approximately 70% of each group rated their health as very good or good at 1 year following the hospitalization.

In summary, the evaluation found that a less costly, less medically intensive Cooperative Care program, emphasizing patient and care partner education, participation in management, and early patient activation, was successfully implemented and well accepted. Further, it demonstrated increased patient understanding, more capable self-management, and better preparation for posthospital care. Patients in Cooperative Care took increased responsibility for their management, and had no adverse outcomes of care. A wide array of patients benefitted.

IMPLICATIONS FOR APPLICATION ELSEWHERE

The experience of the Cooperative Care program and the results of the process and outcome evaluation described above have widespread relevance for the delivery of health services, especially to aging patients and those with chronic diseases, in this country as well as in other Western industrialized countries.

The increasing number and proportion of older individuals contributes significantly to current and projected health care demands and expenditures. The elderly have high rates of chronic diseases which clearly affect morbidity, disability, and use of health services. Such demographic trends and associated health care needs point to the importance of secondary and tertiary prevention for improving the quality of life and maximizing functional capacity in our aging population. All countries experiencing increases in their aging populations have as priorities: 1) the prevention or delay of acute hospitalization and nursing home care, and 2) maintenance of functioning, or at least the retardation of loss of independent functioning. These objectives are aimed at helping to control the costs of health care delivery while improving the quality of life of those affected.

Three specific aspects of Cooperative Care give this model appeal and increase the likelihood of implementation by others in the United States and other industrialized countries: 1) its emphasis on a biopsychosocial model rather than on a strict medical model; 2) the importance of a "significant other" and the family; and 3) the composition and involvement of the health care team who provide treatment, care, and followup for the individual.

Given the shift toward chronic diseases, research and results have shown that the effective treatment of chronic diseases needs to go beyond the usual medical model of "diagnose, treat and cure" to a more comprehensive model, frequently termed the "biopsychosocial model." The biopsychosocial model emphasizes "diagnose, treat and maintain the highest level of independent functioning." This model gives recognition to the fact that many diseases are not curable, particularly chronic diseases that are more prevalent among the aging and the aged. It also emphasizes the importance of social support and environmental factors, which frequently are crucial in the treatment and quality of life of aging individuals who have chronic diseases.

The Cooperative Care program clearly maximizes the involvement of the "significant other"—the family member or friend acting as a care partner—in a unique and innovative way that is not yet common in the delivery of hospital care. Since the early work by Berkman and Syme (1979) and ensuing epidemiological studies and health education interventions, there has been increasing evidence of the importance of a "significant other" or social support in promoting health and preventing disability, as well as in reducing premature death. The key role played by the "significant other" becomes even more important when one considers the fact that most health care occurs at home. Many hospitals, as well as other health care delivery sites, are becoming intensely interested in learning how to include family and friends in order to maximize patient learning, translating this into useful health care behaviors and, in turn, to an improved outcome once the patient returns home.

The involvement of a multiplicity of professionals of differing disciplines in the management and care of patients is also of major importance to the Cooperative Care program and to the results obtained. As noted above, the Cooperative Care group of patients and care partners reported being exposed to more information by more people than those patients receiving routine hospital care. This was associated with increased patient and care partner understanding of the illness and treatment, and their perception that the education they received was helpful in managing the patient's health after discharge. These results clearly point out how useful it is to have different types of professionals involved. Together they can be more instrumental than one professional discipline alone in helping the patient, family, and friends to better manage the care of the patient after discharge from the hospital.

The Cooperative Care program is an innovation in the delivery of health care that is a forerunner in its field. It addresses research and administrative issues. In relation to the landmark work of *Healthy People 2000: The Surgeon General's Report on Health Promotion and Disease Prevention* on meeting health care objectives for the year 2000 (Sullivan, 1990), Cooperative Care stands out as one of the key intervention trials that had already begun to address several of the "priority research areas." These include: 1) the effect of the family on the

health and functional status of elderly people; 2) the characteristics of
the people who are providing care to the elderly; and 3) the impact of
living arrangements on health and functional status. Cooperative
Care can provide many insights regarding areas of health and medical
care delivery that are of top priority. Many institutions also can learn
a great deal from this experience in terms of answering salient and
critical health care research and administrative issues.

In addition to Cooperative Care's applicability throughout the
United States, this experience is extremely pertinent to other Western
industrialized countries that are experiencing similar demographic
trends and health care delivery problems. They, too, have goals of increasing the functional capacity of aging individuals with chronic disease and improving their quality of life. The primary author of this
chapter has been doing research in this area in northern Italy over the
past 4 years and also has participated in an international European
workshop specifically designed to address these issues. There is a
great deal of interest in the implementation of the three major aspects
of the Cooperative Care experience noted above.

Of course, there are specific areas in which differences in experiences between Europe and the United States need to be addressed before cross-cultural transference of this experience can be accomplished. For example, the structure and the physical location of the
family in Europe tends to be much different than in the United States.
Families in Europe tend to live in the same city and area. In Europe,
generations of the same family often live together, or at least are in
close physical proximity, generally living less than 5 miles apart. The
"significant other" for the European is likely to be of a different generation, particularly if the spouse of the patient is no longer living.

The concept of the multidisciplinary professional health care team
as practiced in Cooperative Care is less common in Europe. Due to the
way hospitals currently are structured there, and the training and job
descriptions of the various professionals, the nurse, social worker, and
health educator are often unable or unavailable to perform the tasks
which are jointly accomplished at Cooperative Care. Also, even though
hospitals in Europe are using DRGs and trying to reduce inappropri-
ately long lengths of stay, frequently a hospitalization is used to provide respite care for the family.

These differences should in no way dampen enthusiasm for applying
successful undertakings such as Cooperative Care in different coun-

tries. However, the differences need to be highlighted, understood, and dealt with sensitively by those who are initiating the new program if they are to maximize the positive impact that an effective intervention such as Cooperative Care would bring to their own health care delivery arena.

18

THE REGULATORY ENVIRONMENT OF THE 1970s: NEW YORK UNIVERSITY MEDICAL CENTER'S EXPERIENCE

Irvin G. Wilmot

CONCEPTION

Cooperative Care was conceived in the mid-sixties under a public policy that was widely interpreted by hospital and medical center boards and management teams as "Do more! Do better!" The perceived challenge was to build new and improved patient care services to meet an insatiable public demand. Building a "better mousetrap" was the order of the day and, for the most part, hospitals nationwide focused on fulfilling that policy expectation. Retrospective cost reimbursement and widening entitlements, both public and private, enhanced and fueled the process.

In 1964, New York University Medical Center had reached a near impasse in its operation, with no unoccupied "cold beds" other than those on the pediatric and obstetric services. Without being labelled as "emergent"—the accuracy of such labelling was monitored by the department chairman via the chief medical resident—it was nearly impossible to achieve a spot on the medical waiting list for admission. The earliest preoperative booking on the surgical schedule loomed many weeks ahead. All of this occurred, strangely enough, only 18 months after the institution had moved into a totally new replacement hospital which was sized 60% larger than its 90-year-old, 387–bed predecessor. Under these circumstances, with an energetic clinical faculty as its medical staff, and with a receptive board of trustees, bed expansion seemed in order.

The original planning focus for the new beds was, indeed, "Do better!" At the outset, cost considerations were very much lower in priority than creating an improved product. However, cost gained more importance as the project evolved. The major objective of the project was to overcome some of the difficulties and shortcomings of the patient's experience in the traditional inpatient setting. Five such deficiencies were identified:

1. noninvolvement of family in the care of patients in the hospital;
2. inadequate preparation of patients for postdischarge management of chronic disease;
3. inefficient and high-cost logistics of the hospital's diagnostic, treatment, and hotel-like services;
4. unnecessary capital expenditure for physical plant features and standards which were unneeded for particular types of admissions or for portions of certain hospitalizations; and
5. inappropriate "sickroom" environment for recuperative patients who should be learning to readjust to a healthier role.

With the caveat that the new facility would serve acute care patients *only*, overcoming or ameliorating these negatives became the goal, and formed the roots from which Cooperative Care emerged. Management of the medical center, including nursing, formed the nucleus of the planning group. Presented with the concept, the group enthusiastically embraced the new venture and, with the input of physicians and other professionals, quickly developed generalized operating principles and preliminary procedures. To arrive at the right-sized unit, the patient population of the hospital was surveyed with the newly developed admission criteria of the proposed project in mind. Tentative financing was arranged and architectural schematics developed. The governing body said "Go," and management set out for the tedious arenas of regulation and reimbursement.

REGULATORY CLIMATE

In the 15 years between Cooperative Care's conception and completion (1964–1979), hospitals in New York State experienced an unsettling swing in regulatory climate. On the payment front, a' movement from retrospective cost reimbursement to state-controlled (Medicare excepted) all-payor rates occurred. As might be expected, the swing was less a smooth fluid arc and more a wavering, back-and-forth action. The period was fraught with constant change. New rules seemed to arrive daily. It was an environment which was unpredictable even by the rulemakers. It was a difficult time for budget projections and financial planning for normal operations, let alone for an atypical venture like Cooperative Care.

During the same period, the certificate of need process moved from being a voluntary, privately financed regional planning mechanism to a legislated, formal, state-managed and -financed process. Cooperative Care received one of the last certificates of need granted by the Regional Planning Council. The certificate of need remained valid throughout the project's life, thanks not only to its merit, but also to a combination of political perseverance and sheer good fortune. That still left licensure and reimbursement as the major regulatory hurdles to be overcome.

In 1969, in the name of cost containment, legislation was passed empowering the state health commissioner to assure the "efficient production of hospital services." With the same penstroke, Blue Cross payment rates were coupled to those for Medicaid, and the state moved slowly toward a single rate-setting methodology. The new responsibilities of the Department of Health were enormous, and its assumption of those responsibilities a multiyear process. The flux described continued through the day of dedication for the project.

One major policy of the new order significantly affected reimbursement and licensure negotiations. This was a bed reduction policy and program implemented by the State Department of Health early in its new life. Based upon data and the commissioner's belief, which was shared by many, that New York was grossly overbedded with unjustifiable and unexplainably high lengths of stay, a statewide bed reduction program sprung to life. Within 2 years more than 40 hospitals closed their doors and a freeze on new bed additions was imposed. The Cooperative Care certificate of need, authorizing new beds, acquired a new value overnight and became a fair target for zealous bureaucrats inside and outside of government. Fortunately for the project, senior regulators had open minds, embraced the concept in varying degrees and, in the end, tried hard to find a niche for Cooperative Care in their view of the law and their responsibilities.

LICENSURE AND REIMBURSEMENT

Licensure as an acute care facility was an imperative. Cooperative Care was to incur all of the cost of providing the full range of hospital diagnostic and therapeutic services, and required corollary reimbursement. The two most difficult propositions for regulators and reimbursers to accept were the notions of substitutive rather than additive days and the reality that Cooperative Care patients, in fact, would be "hospital sick." A full description of the quantity and character of the dialogue on these issues is not possible within the limits of this volume. It was lengthy, it was frequent, and it seemed endless; but it did produce results. Formal recognition of Cooperative Care's acute care status came on the operating certificate, which arrived shortly before opening day. A discrete category within the acute care classification was awarded the facility. This was, indeed, an appropriate and satisfactory outcome.

During the period of development and construction of the project, the roles and authority of the nonfederal rate-setters was not crystal clear. These third-party payors, the Department of Health's Office of Health Systems Management (OHSM) and Blue Cross, were working through their respective roles in the new scheme of a fully regulated hospital environment. OHSM, in its early stages of development both within and without, faced many issues on many fronts. Blue Cross was resisting its loss of power and, with discrete rates and benefit packages still intact, strived to conduct business as usual. It should be noted, however, that the commercial insurers were not players at that time. By simply indemnifying their policyholders against hospital expense, they acquired no voice. Medicare, which was providing 35% of the admissions to the hospital, and Blue Cross, which had 80% of the hospital insurance market share in the metropolitan area, were the important payors. They were the ones who would determine financial viability of the project. Negotiations with both parties were begun.

The regional office of Medicare embraced the concept of Cooperative Care. It was enthusiastic about the project, but lacked the necessary authority to establish rates or approve the sort of modification to traditional hospital care being proposed. Jurisdiction resided in Washington, where support for the concept was forthcoming, not with the same ebullience displayed in the region, but with genuine interest. Inclusion of the costs of the care partner in the reimbursement rate was troublesome for Medicare. The hospital argued that the costs for the care partner would be smaller than those incurred in a traditional setting for similar but lesser service and, further, that patients would not choose Cooperative Care if out-of-pocket expense were necessary. A number of trips to Baltimore, followed by a period of deliberation by Medicare, yielded approval of Cooperative Care as a "demonstration project" with acute care rates. It was agreed that a formal objective evaluation was to be undertaken before a final subsequent assessment was made.

Blue Cross was troubled by the same issues that bothered Medicare. Most particularly, Blue Cross was concerned that days in Cooperative Care would be additive to the length of stay. This was a problem because hospital reimbursement at that time was on a per diem basis. Discussions similar to those held at the federal level ensued, and concurrence finally was reached. Blue Cross decided that it would accept Cooperative Care beds as acute beds, thereby including them in both benefit packages and reimbursement rates. "Demonstration" and "evaluation" qualifiers, as with Medicare, were the quid pro quo. A deal you say? Not quite! The "quid" for Blue Cross had one more "quo."

Anxious to aid the cause of bed reduction and establish a reputation of wise and prudent oversight, Blue Cross demanded an additional contingent condition. The hospital would be required to find and remove from the state's total bed inventory a number of acute care beds equal to the number of Cooperative Care beds to be built. OHSM readily joined the "hardball game" as either a partner or supporter. At this point the distinction between those terms was immaterial. Thus, the hospital began its search for available obsolete beds.

Historically, hospital development in New York City over the years included many very small (under 75 beds) institutions. Most of these had started as proprietary ventures in order to fill an unmet local need, and they were converted into community nonprofit institutions in later years. The burgeoning technology of modern medicine and the inefficiency of their small size made for obsolescence and financial distress. One such 60-bed institution in midtown Manhattan was identified and an expression of merger interest solicited. The timing was right. The administrator of many years was nearing retirement and the governing body was uneasy about the future.

The target hospital, a merger policy set, brought a second large institution, which was more favored by their medical staff, into the competition. Its major interest was the liquidated value, mostly real estate, of the institution. NYU's interest was primarily the beds available. The forays, feints, and intrigue that followed is the stuff of novels. The decision turned, finally, on which of the merger suitors was willing to keep the existing hospital operating for an additional 2 years, as that was the sentimental desire of the retiring executive. Faced with this requirement, the competition withdrew and NYU, for a 2-year period, had one more hospital to manage. Negotiations with OHSM won a two-for-one bed credit, giving NYU a 120–bed credit balance. Cooperative Care consumed 104 of those beds; the remainder were used to offset bed reduction requirements for a freestanding ambulatory surgical unit which was under concurrent development. Society was well served. Cooperative Care began its life and Blue Cross closed one more outmoded, unneeded hospital without the political onus of direct action.

In its years of operation, Cooperative Care has thrived in an ever-changing regulatory atmosphere. DRGs have replaced per diem payments, average lengths of stay have nosedived; "hospital-sick" is different from what it was; and total quality management (TQM) has overtaken utilization review. Although evaluation continues as an ongoing good management practice, the "demonstration" label is long gone; Cooperative Care is "acute hospital care," and fully recognized as such. It seems certain that, as the 1990s proceed, more regulatory change will come. Cooperative Care, along with other care modalities, will need to establish and justify its role in the nation's evolving search for quality, cost-effective, accessible health services.

THE PLANNING PROCESS

NYU Medical Center in the 1960s and 1970s enjoyed a stability and organizational comfort of a high order. Strong mutual trust prevailed among the governing body, the faculty, the staff, and executive management. All were joined in a common effort to advance the Medical Center's interests. Of course, differences among individuals and constituencies, as are present in all complex organizations, did occur.

Most, however, were either resolved or an agreement reached to disagree. Seldom were they left to fester. This resulted in a climate which was most conducive to productive effort.

Planning for Cooperative Care was not a single focus effort. The structure which was to be built would contain programs for faculty practice offices (physician's offices), ambulatory surgery suites, a radiological imaging center, an outpatient laboratory, and an outpatient pharmacy, in addition to Cooperative Care. This circumstance tended to spread constituency interest among the various program elements. Information checkpoints for the Board of Trustees and for the medical staff were scheduled throughout the planning process. A few physicians developed a genuine interest in the Cooperative Care concept and provided valuable input.

For the most part, the majority of the medical staff viewed the Cooperative Care project as representing 104 additional and much needed beds. They felt that those beds would be convertible in the future, if necessary, to traditional hospital beds. Management's dilemma was whether to attempt to force an understanding of the concept before the fact, or to produce the product first with understanding to follow. The latter option was chosen and planning proceeded quietly, yet in the open, with full disclosure of the unique features of the new beds. To what extent this course contributed to the initial marketing difficulties with the medical staff once the unit was opened is not known. The consensus is "some, but not a lot." In summary, the program planning was carried on by a small group of people with frequent professional staff consultation. It was free of "turf tussles" and other distractions, with almost no second-thought "if onlys" upon completion.

There was little direct participation of external parties in the actual detailed planning process of the program itself. Other than seeking endorsement and approval for the certificate of need, licensure, and reimbursement, the Medical Center did not solicit external involvement in program planning, nor did interested parties force their participation. The single state-imposed requirement was that the Medical Center plan for an alternate use of the facility in the event that the Cooperative Care concept failed. Economic and political prudence supported such a "back door" exit for state officials and hospital management alike. Architectural feasibility and schematic plans for possible future economic conversion of patient floors to a nursing home use were developed and, likely, gather dust to this day.

A final historical note for the curious: The abnormal 15 year gestation of Cooperative Care was the product of two factors: the unpredictability of the regulatory changes and reimbursement patterns in New York State throughout the period, and a precipitous action of Blue

Cross. Hospital managements throughout the state were constantly attempting to cope with the regulatory and reimbursement changes. NYU was no exception, as it struggled to maintain existing services and was wary of new, high-risk ventures. Each change in the ground rules reinforced anxiety and, although experience and time mitigated concern, uncertainty was always present. In retrospect, the thousands of individual regulatory mandates of the period blur into a single movement toward full regulation of hospitals in New York State. Each individual rule, at the time, lacked that perspective, and was viewed as having the potential for producing real damage to the individual institutions.

An arbitrary action by Blue Cross reducing reimbursement for capital expenditure to 50 cents on the dollar occurred as the initial program was going to bid. The edict was ill-conceived and short-lived, but served to cool the eagerness to build by many degrees. This setback, together with a high preliminary cost projection for the project, prompted redesign and relocation to an alternate site. While the original program for the project was well conceived, it contained elements of excess, such as a plush recreational area for the professional staff, which were not compatible with emerging economic realities. The elongated gestation gave birth to an enhanced product, innovative in terms of patient care and viable not only in the economics of the day, but in the years to follow.

19

ADAPTING THE CONCEPT TO A SMALL UNIT: THE VERMONT EXPERIENCE

Rosemary Dale

MOTIVATION

The Medical Center Hospital of Vermont (MCHV), in Burlington, Vermont, is a 550–bed secondary and tertiary care facility. The MCHV offers a full range of services and is centrally located on the campus of the University of Vermont. The medical staff is an open one, accommodating full-time university physicians and part-time community physicians. Patients are drawn from a broad area, which encompasses all of Vermont and a portion of northern New York.

Despite its bucolic placement, MCHV is prey to the same forces which have affected all health care facilities during the past decade. In 1985, as we attempted to analyze and deal with these forces, we became motivated to consider the idea of adapting Cooperative Care to our area. This concept was appealing as a less expensive, more desirable way to provide care to a select group of patients. We further felt that implementation of such a plan might help us respond to some of the pressures of competition, consumerism and finance that were affecting us so heavily.

ADVANTAGES: "SUDS"

As we began our exploration of the Cooperative Care concept, the advantages that surfaced seemed to cluster in four areas. We created the acronym "SUDS" to depict these areas. Our equation was: *S*avings + *U*se of staff + *D*ischarge readiness = *S*atisfaction.

With regard to the first item, savings, we felt that we could run the unit at significantly less cost than a routine care bed. This would be accomplished by transferring as many tasks as possible to the patient or care partner, thus cutting down on the number of personnel required in the unit.

The second item was use of staff. If we achieved our first goal, not only would we achieve cost reduction, but we would free the professional staff for activities such as patient and family assessment, patient teaching, and early discharge planning. Thus, we had a dual goal: to reduce the number of hospital-paid personnel, and to provide a stimulating environment in which professionals would feel that their talents were being maximized.

The third item was discharge readiness. We felt that by having the patient and care partner participate in every aspect of care from the beginning of the hospitalization, we would demystify the disease process for them, thereby having them become more comfortable with the disease and its management. By effecting this demystification and education, we expected earlier discharge.

The sum of these three items—the savings that would be achieved from use of fewer personnel, the use of staff in a professionally satisfying way, and the creation of earlier discharge readiness—seemed to add up to a broad satisfaction for all involved: the hospital, staff, and patients, as well as the physicians admitting to the unit.

RISK ISSUES

In February, 1985, an administrative decision was made to implement Cooperative Care on a trial basis. The decision was based on establishing a situation that would produce minimal risk to the hospital. We looked at risk as having four major issues: 1) capital and startup operational funds; 2) staffing; 3) reimbursement; and 4) regulatory agencies.

The first risk issue was capital and start-up operational funds. We put a $10 thousand ceiling on the funds that would be allotted to this project. The space identified for Cooperative Care was a vacant eight-bed area that had been previously used as a coronary care unit. It would require no major renovation for conversion to its new use. The mentality "use as is" was a keynote of developing this project.

The second risk issue was staffing. We would employ no incremental staff. The assessment was made that the Cooperative Care Unit would not increase patient volume for MCHV, but rather would displace patients who otherwise would have been on the routine care units.

The third risk issue was reimbursement. We met with the local Blue Cross/Blue Shield plan as well as with Medicare representatives to explain the project and to indicate that admission to the Cooperative Care Unit would be limited to those patients who are eligible for acute care hospitalization. This would not be a hotel facility or an area to house patients who required less than acute hospital care. We agreed that during the first 6 months of the project, each patient to be admitted to Cooperative Care would undergo a preadmission utilization review assessment.

The fourth risk area was the regulatory agencies, particularly the State Department of Health. Since the unit did not increase the total number of beds in the institution, we were not subjected to Certificate of Need regulations. We also reviewed the policies of the new unit with our liability insurer to avoid any surprises for either party in the event that a litigious situation arose in the future.

PATIENT SELECTION

With risk assessment completed, we were ready to move ahead and select a manager for the area. Our feeling was that selection of this individual would be one of the most important moves our institution could make in determining the success or failure of the new unit. We selected a nurse-clinician who had been with MCHV for 5 years and had a strong background in general medical/surgical nursing, particularly in cardiovascular disease. At this juncture, we turned over formulation of day-to-day policies, the task of marketing, and the actual preparation of the unit to the new manager.

One of the first activities at this point was to set up a patient selection process. In order for a patient to enter the Cooperative Care Unit, the attending physician would need to grade this unit as an acceptable placement. Subsequently, the nurse-clinician would interview the patient to determine whether their nursing care needs could be met in this environment. Of course, the patient would have to be willing to be in this setting.

Early in our planning, we naively used four qualifications for admission to Cooperative Care: 1) the patient had to be ambulatory; 2) the patient would require minimal nursing care; 3) the patient would have a care partner available; and 4) the patient would qualify for hospitalization. By August, 1986, our understanding had matured, and we simplified our admission qualifications to just one question: "Can the patient safely receive care in the Cooperative Care Unit?" We currently include patients who are nonambulatory and who do not have care partners, and we no longer prescreen for qualification for hospitalization.

Since the inception of the new unit, our entire institution, like others throughout the country, handles sicker and sicker patients. The walking-well patients we had initially hoped for no longer exist in our hospital. Our ability to adapt to a sicker population throughout the institution requires more nursing intervention, so with its reduced staffing needs Cooperative Care remains quite attractive to us.

NUTS AND BOLTS

Having worked out a patient selection process, the next issue faced by the manager was what we call the "nuts and bolts" of the unit. Eight items were identified:

- *The emergency call system.* How would patients in Cooperative Care get in touch with nursing personnel when they needed assistance? A telephone was placed in each patient room, and the hospital operator would page the nursing supervisor if no nurse were in attendance on the unit.
- *The self-medication policy.* We formulated a homelike distribution system so that patients would be provided bulk medications rather than unit-dose packaging. The purpose of this plan was for effectiveness of education, as we wanted patients to receive their medications the same way they would from a commercial pharmacy.
- Transportation. How would we get patients to and from the vari-

ous areas of the medical center? We decided to use care partners and hospital staff escorts.

- Charting. With nursing staff on the unit only during certain hours, some charting would fall to the patient and care partner.
- Dress code. We would encourage patients in the unit to wear street clothes.
- Patient identification. We decided to use an arm band as we do for the rest of the medical center.
- The fire plan. We put clear instructions in every room regarding how to report a fire and how to evacuate the area in an emergency.
- Nursing assistance. We would initially provide 8 hours of nursing care per day on the unit. However, as the unit became busier, we lengthened the nursing coverage to 12.5 hours per day.

PROBLEMS

Initially, one of our greatest concerns was how to handle patients who do not have care partners. However, as more experience was gained in operating the unit, the nurse-clinician became able to identify those patients who can safely be managed without a care partner in attendance. We worried as well about anxiety developing over the responsibility faced by the care partner overnight, with the nursing supervisor only making rounds every two or three hours. As a corollary, we worried about patients who would have unpredictable courses; for example, someone experiencing chest pain during the night. We decided that if the situation warranted, we would move the patient from Cooperative Care into a more traditional medical/surgical unit bed. As we became more knowledgeable about the process, we have had very few inaccurate assessments. Patients and care partners who do not want to share responsibility for their care, or who are not adequately prepared for one reason or another, would fall into the category of poor assessment. The number of moves to a traditional bed because of undue anxiety, an unpredictable course, or poor assessment have been very few.

STATISTICS

Patients are fairly evenly split between male and female, and range in age from infancy to 88 years. Care partners, the majority of whom are women (mainly mothers or wives) range in age from 21 to 74 years. The most frequent categories of patients encountered have been cardiology, ophthalmology, pediatrics, oncology, radiation therapy, burns, and renal transplant recipients.

Early in the operation of the unit we became aware that the average length of stay in Cooperative Care for each DRG was significantly lower than the national average. Patient and care partner satisfaction has been high.

CONCLUSION

In conclusion, adapting Cooperative Care to a small unit can be successful. It can limit some portion of health care costs. It can engender demonstrably high levels of consumer satisfaction and enhance an institution's position in a competitive market. It can serve as a model of change and flexibility within an institution. Finally, implementation of such a unit, with sharing of care responsibilities with patients and their families, can be viewed as a strong statement by the institution about the direction of health care it foresees for the future.

PART II
The Cooperative Care Center of Rhode Island: A Center in Development

Health policy has done a complete turnaround in the 15 years since the New York University Medical Center's Cooperative Care Center opened. Although regulation remains prevalent, especially with regard to certificates of need for construction, the Reagan and Bush eras brought competition to the health care marketplace. This phenomenon occurred at about the time that prospective payment became universal for recipients of Medicare, a trend rapidly being adopted by Blue Cross plans and even some commercial insurers around the country. The prepaid care movement began to grow, too. These forces resulted in a major shift of emphasis away from inpatient care to outpatient/ambulatory care, leaving hospitals, often with considerable excess bed capacity, scrambling for increasingly small pieces of the inpatient pie.

This part of the book describes the planning for the Cooperative Care Center of Rhode Island, the second large-scale cooperative care unit in the United States. This 74–bed Center, which is under construction at the time of this writing and scheduled to open in July 1994, is modeled on the NYU Center, but with several major adaptations.

The goal of the new center is to provide academic medical center quality of care at community hospital prices. The most significant difference between the New York and Rhode Island centers is that the latter is a joint venture between two hospitals, Rhode Island Hospital and Women and Infants Hospital. Further, as a reflection of changing times and market forces at work, there is a strong emphasis on guest relations and the amenities of care. In fact, Marriott Health Care Services will manage the hospitality functions. This partnership brings with it a strong service quality initiative that has long been important in the hotel industry and is only recently being adopted in health care facilities.

Concomitant with the focus on hospitality is a strong emphasis on marketing the Cooperative Care Center of Rhode Island, not merely within the state but in Connecticut and Massachusetts as well. This, again is a reflection of changing times. Other anticipated differences include the diagnostic mix and the delivery of nursing services. All of these proposed changes are discussed in detail in the pages that follow.

Because of Rhode Island's limited geographic boundaries, Providence, the state's capital, is actually a city-state with a population of approximately 1 million people. It is located about 40 miles southeast of Boston and 100 miles northeast of New Haven, both major medical centers. The Cooperative Care Center of Rhode Island expects to compete in these geographic areas.

20

WHY RHODE ISLAND HOSPITAL CHOSE COOPERATIVE CARE

Bruce K. Komiske

Health care reform is here. Its impact on the construction of inpatient beds is significant. Hospitals will continue to need to replace old and inefficient inpatient facilities, but the actual number of beds has decreased in most institutions, and the impact of managed care is likely to further this decline. Therefore, an opportunity exists to do things differently, and not merely replace traditional beds.

Gone are the days when the cost of replacement facilities was reimbursed through debt service and depreciation expense passed on as part of the cost of doing business. Gone are days of easy access to tax-exempt debt based on strong hospital bond ratings. These changes already have made a significant difference in the mindsets of hospital administrators around the country who have had active projects in the planning stage totaling billions of dollars. They now are very concerned about the impact these additional costs may have in a managed care environment where hospitals convert from being profit centers to cost centers. These changes create significant challenges, as the institutions will be forced to compete from service, quality, and cost perspectives in this new era.

Rhode Island Hospital (RIH), a 719-bed academic medical center, is the largest comprehensive care facility in the state and the primary teaching hospital of Brown University School of Medicine. In 1993, the hospital is running an average length of stay of 6.3 days and an average percent occupancy in the low 80s. Except for obstetrics and neonatology, which are services provided by Women and Infants Hospital (WIH), Rhode Island Hospital is a full line/full service institution, with a 23% market share in the state. Its physical plant consists of approximately 1.2 million square feet in 23 buildings located on its 52–acre urban campus.

In the late 1980s, as a result of a Campus Master Plan process, Rhode Island Hospital was forced to address its need to replace its aging physical plant. Its inpatient bed facilities averaged 40 years of continuous service, with roughly 70% of the beds located in four-bed rooms which lacked some basic hospital amenities. As one of the founders of a health care network and a growing PPO, the hospital also began to recognize its need to compete on both a cost as well as a quality basis, not only with the tertiary centers in Boston, but also with some of the community hospitals in its own state.

Through its strategic planning process and a renewed interest in service, the hospital also identified the need to listen to its customers and demonstrate value to patients, their employers and third-party payors. It was this combination of factors that led the institution to look externally for other models of inpatient care which could positively impact on both cost and quality.

At the same time, Women and Infants Hospital, the State's major provider of obstetrical and neonatal services, with nearly 10,000 births annually and 66% of the state's obstetrics market share, had recently moved to the Rhode Island Hospital campus. WIH had the good fortune of a beautiful new 137-bed facility. However, with an average occupancy rate that was well above 90%, and many days exceeding 100% capacity of existing beds, WIH had become a victim of its own success.

While both hospitals share the same campus and originally had major expectations of improved efficiency through shared services, little progress had been made in actually developing cooperative efforts to achieve economies of scale. While the objectives of each institution were somewhat different, the leadership of each hospital decided that the time was right to join forces in the development of a new facility to serve their respective goals.

Rather than build more traditional beds, given the changes on the horizon, an effort was made to seek out the best practices occurring throughout the country, especially alternatives to traditional hospital construction. Staff members from both hospitals traveled to the Hospital/Hotel at Abbott Northwestern, Minneapolis, MN, a hotel on an academic medical center campus which accommodates patients who come from far away and where some outpatient services are provided; the Temple Medical Center-Medical Inn in New Haven, a hotel with minimal medical assistance available, where patients can recover from surgery or diagnostic procedures; and the Planetree Unit in California. This latter unit provides a patient-focused environment through architecture and patient education. None of these approaches, however, provides any substantial cost savings. It was not until the group visited the NYU Cooperative Care Center that they felt they had seen a model which satisfactorily demonstrated lower cost and enhanced quality. At that time, the NYU unit had been in operation for 8 years.

The initial visit with NYU started an ongoing dialogue with key staff from both Rhode Island Hospital and Women and Infants Hospital with the NYU staff which, as of 1993, spanned a 6-year period of encouragement and support. The remaining chapters of this book describe the issues, plans, and dreams of the RIH and WIH staff, as we anticipate the opening of the Cooperative Care Center of Rhode Island. We hope and pray that it will meet our high expectations, and look forward to an opportunity to share our experience with the health care community after we become fully operational.

21

REGULATORY AND FINANCIAL ISSUES FACED BY RHODE ISLAND'S CENTER

Robert F. Menard, Bruce K. Komiske, and Kenneth Weiner

The health care industry is extremely conservative, and hospitals are among the more conservative components of the system. From its inception, most hospital reimbursement under Medicare was based on retrospective cost formulas which provided little or no incentive for hospitals to contain costs. It was only with the implementation of DRG reimbursement in 1986 that hospitals were pressured to seek out ways of becoming more cost-effective in order to survive. Even with this change, appropriate "pass-throughs" were made for capital expenditures through proportionate sharing of costs for depreciation and interest expense.

Frustration with lack of financial incentives and innovation in the health care industry was shared by many. It was particularly well articulated by Dr. David Axelrod, former Commissioner of Health for the State of New York. In a speech given at a conference on cooperative care in 1989, Dr. Axelrod chastised hospitals in general by commenting from his role as final approval authority for certificates of need in the State:

> Hospitals spend billions of dollars a year on new facilities which have not significantly changed their basic design over the past 30 years. The "box" in which the beds are located has been modified from a cross concept to a circular concept, to a rectangular concept, to a double-loaded corridor concept and more currently, to a pod concept. The reality, however, is that not one of the proposed bed plans has been able to significantly demonstrate any operating savings in the provision of care. . .

Dr. Axelrod, who was an initial skeptic of the cooperative care concept, then continued:

> For the first time in the history of hospitals as we know them today, the cooperative care concept is based on the ability to provide quality inpatient care at a lower cost. (D. Axelrod, unpublished data).

It is easy to appreciate Dr. Axelrod's comments. However, when a hospital administrator is faced with the prospect of replacing antiquated beds and can go forward with a time tested traditional approach which would be questioned by few or, as an alternative, propose implementing a concept that has only been used once, the incentives are not yet sufficiently strong for administrators and boards to take the risk.

In 1987, Rhode Island Hospital and Women and Infants Hospital took the risk and formed a joint venture to build a medical inn as part of a "Medical Mall" on the campus which they share in South Providence. A certificate of need was approved by the Health Planning Council, but regulators were uncertain as to how to classify these nontraditional beds and, therefore, were unwilling to issue a hospital license for the medical inn. At the same time, however, they expected the inn to function as part of the hospital in terms of bearing its proportionate share of charitable allowances and bad debts.

Blue Cross, as a participant in the CON approval process, determined that it was unwilling to reimburse the medical inn until after it was operational, given the fact that it lacked a hospital license for acute care. This created a catch-22 situation. Without a license there was no guarantee of reimbursement; without reimbursement, there was no way to demonstrate success of a lower-care alternative to tradi-tional inpatient beds. In the end, the trustees of both institutions de-cided that, if they were to proceed with the new venture, it would have to be with assurance of reimbursement and, therefore, the project would have to be approved as licensed hospital beds.

In 1990, Rhode Island Hospital (RIH) and Women and Infants Hospi-tal (WIH) filed a new certificate of need to build the Cooperative Care Center of Rhode Island, a facility modeled after that developed by NYU. By then, the State Health Planning Council had issued a mora-torium on the construction of new hospital beds, a moratorium which remains in effect at the time of this writing. For Rhode Island Hospi-tal this did not present a problem, since its portion of the Cooperative Care beds (81% or 60 beds) were to serve as replacement beds for out-moded ones in the main hospital.

For Women and Infants Hospital, the need was completely different. Women and Infants was consistently operating at greater than 100% capacity anywhere from 3 to 10 days a month. That put it out of com-pliance with its operating license and, despite the moratorium, cre-ated a demand that it expand capacity in order to comply with other health department regulations.

The Certificate of Need application indicated that the Cooperative Care Center would see a fairly representative cross-section of the cur-rent inpatient population for both institutions, as well as an unquanti-fiable number of patients who would otherwise be admitted for tradi-tional hospital care at other acute care hospitals in Rhode Island or the neighboring states of Massachusetts and Connecticut.

In an attempt to stretch limited hospital capital, the Cooperative Care Center was originally to have been financed by the builder/devel-oper. However, it became apparent that the cost of capital would be as much as two percentage points higher than if the money were to be ac-quired under tax-exempt bonds. Further, the developer would require a long-term master lease, which in essence would guarantee payment of the loan. Thus, the hospitals decided that it would be better to pro-ceed on their own. As a result, construction is being financed through a combination of owner's equity and the sale of $10.6 million of 30–year bonds issued by the Rhode Island Health and Educational Build-ing Corporation. Excluding the value of the land, which is owned by Rhode Island Hospital, the debt is being shared at 81% RIH and 19% WIH.

To give further comfort to the boards of both RIH and WIH, a finan-cial feasibility study was undertaken by KPMG Peat Marwick in 1990. It concluded that sufficient funds could be generated to meet the Cooperative Care Center of Rhode Island's annual operating expense and other financial requirements, including the debt service requirements associated with the construction, given the reimbursement structure which existed at the time. The report went on to recommend that the hospitals address the following issues, if they were to achieve success:

1. An educational and marketing plan for the hospital's medical staff, insurance payors, and community had to be developed, specifically stating the advantages of the cooperative care concept. Pivotal to this program is the identification of a physician "champion" to lead the effort.

2. Within the overall hospital market plan, market share targets for the cooperative care facility had to be developed, with a management action plan to achieve the targets.

3. Through patient surveys, the hospital needed to identify the availability of care partners for the market segments to be considered appropriate for the cooperative care concept.

The report concluded that, although the need for a cooperative care facility was more one of capacity for Women and Infants Hospital and replacement of antiquated facilities for Rhode Island Hospital, both hospitals must position the new facility in a volatile marketplace in which its clinical and financial advantages are understood and accepted.

The Health Planning Council approved the second CON and the health department issued a license to operate the center as a hospital. However, one of the Health Planning Council's conditions of approval of the CON for the Cooperative Care Center was the specification that the charge-per-day be $140 less than for traditional care at Rhode Island Hospital and $70 less for Women and Infants Hospital. The hospitals are optimistic that they can meet these conditions, given the significant impact that Cooperative Care will have on both construction and operating costs.

Average construction costs per square foot for various types of facilities in Rhode Island are: Marriott Inn $75, nursing home $85, acute care hospital $180. The Cooperative Care construction costs are $126 per square foot. The reason for these significant savings over a typical acute care facility will be discussed in greater detail in the architectural and design chapter.

From an operating cost perspective, the Cooperative Care Center of Rhode Island also anticipates its ability to demonstrate significant savings similar to those achieved by NYU. As of the summer of 1993, an operating budget has been prepared which dramatically demonstrates the impact of care partners, particularly on nursing staffing. Although it is difficult to present a perfect "apples to apples" comparison in staffing costs between cooperative care and traditional care, the management engineer assigned to the project has estimated the total personnel costs per patient, compared with traditional care, to be approximately 30% lower for the Cooperative Care unit, including management, clinical staff, hospitality and fringe benefits.

As a result of both significantly lower capital and operating costs, Rhode Island Hospital anticipates that it will be able to replace 60 of its aging inpatient beds in a new and attractive facility, with the total costs, including debt service and depreciation, equaling its existing cost to operate its 40–year-old beds. This assumes 20% equity in the project and does not include the cost of land.

Only time and proper postoccupancy evaluation will determine the ultimate success of this venture. However, as we look to the future, we are hopeful that, with a second major facility of its kind in existence, and a clear demonstration of the Cooperative Care Center's ability to provide quality inpatient care at significantly lower construction and operating costs, there will be a renewed interest in this innovative alternative. We also are optimistic that, with significant reforms in the payment system for health care, appropriate financial incentives will be incorporated to encourage further experimentation and innovation, not just for the cooperative care concept, but for other models as well.

22

ARCHITECTURAL AND DESIGN CONSIDERATIONS

James R. Carlson, David S. Frieder,
Diane Hanley, Rosalyn Cama, and Richard Kuehl

THE BEGINNING

The architect's first task was site selection and master planning for
the medical mall. Rhode Island Hospital had recently acquired an adjoining industrial property which it intended to use for this facility.
Preliminary studies concluded that the site was sufficient in land area
and well suited for the intended purpose. For example, it would be possible to connect to the heart of the existing hospital via an elevated
bridge, with access to the main operating room facilities, and there
would be adequate space for adjacent parking. These master planning
studies identified that the site would also support the approximately
30,000 square feet required to relocate an aging 20-year-old ambulatory surgery center to the medical mall project, further creating syner-
gies among all three components.

A unique aspect, from the architect's design standpoint, is the joint involvement of two separate hospitals, Rhode Island Hospital (RIH) and Women and Infants Hospital (WIH). The two hospitals established internal guidelines for their relationship during this process. For the architect, it meant two clients, acting in concert at times, but with different constituencies and goals. With three buildings in one—the Cooperative Care Center, Ambulatory Surgical Unit and Medical Office Building—and two hospitals with a developer, the number and size of meetings exploded.

PROGRAM DEVELOPMENT

The program development approach chosen by RIH/WIH was designed to be very open and interactive, both among staff and between staff and consultants. The program committee had co-chairmen, one from each institution. Subcommittees, with representation from each hospital, were formed to address each component of the Cooperative Care Center, such as food service, facility management, administration, education, nursing, and medical staff.

Since the Cooperative Care Center of Rhode Island is based on the New York University Medical Center's Cooperative Care model, the process began with an in-depth review of the NYU model. The architects visited the facility with committee members on numerous occasions to review both the physical plant and its operation. At that time, the NYU unit had been in operation for 10 years. Although it had undergone program changes, there had been almost no physical plant changes, except in food service and admitting. Space in admitting, education, and treatment areas appeared to be taxed by the present operation. The patient floor areas at the NYU Cooperative Care Center had functioned well over the 10 year period with no substantial changes being made.

NYU has observed over the years that, as in hospitals across the country, their patients have become more critically ill and more frail. RIH/WIH analyzed their present patient profile and identified those who would qualify for the Cooperative Care Center. This analysis concluded that patient care spanned a wide variety of treatment and age groups. It was concluded that children would not be included as patients, their care being more suited to the new Hasbro Children's Hospital which will incorporate many program elements of Cooperative Care.

The committees all concluded that the space to be allocated for the treatment areas in the new Cooperative Care Center was most critical.

To this end, the NYU space allocation was analyzed, comparing it on a per-patient basis to the planned Cooperative Care Center of Rhode Island. Each independent committee analyzed its proposed services and, in turn, the spaces required to support those services. The architect applied this input and investigated potential conflicts as well as opportunities to share spaces, functions, or activities. Cooperative care encourages the development of cross-trained, multidisciplinary staff. Staffing must be given very early consideration, as staff size and function has a direct impact on the architecture. This is the most significant area in which savings in operational staff and organization translates to initial construction cost savings by defining programmed space accurately.

Cooperative Care is similar to other medical design projects in that future change is inevitable. Spaces must be designed to be as flexible as possible, and the architecture and engineering must anticipate and allow for these changes. Future growth is one such issue and it was programmed into the Cooperative Care Center. Twenty-four additional patient beds were programmed for the future, and treatment areas were programmed to suit an ultimate size of 100 beds. Present bed construction was limited to 74. Allocation of new beds in Rhode Island was considered unattainable through the Certificate of Need process, hence the Cooperative Care Center is the result of replacing existing outdated four-bed rooms at Rhode Island Hospital.

In planning for possible later expansion, treatment areas were given program priority. Some horizontal expansion was considered most desirable. The adjoining medical office building space, along with the south terrace, provides this flexibility. Rentable office space initially will occupy the area programmed for possible future additional beds.

The program planning effort identified five areas of patient treatment or support:

1. Admission/discharge/patient services;
2. Administration;
3. Education;
4. Treatment/close observation; and
5. Support areas: food service/dining/housekeeping

Review of the NYU space allocation, the RIH/WIH patient profile analysis, and committee input established the program listing of spaces and established sizes of spaces. Most discussion and concern centered around the sizes of treatment facilities, admitting spaces and numbers of observation beds required. The admitting/discharge process and the required architectural spaces for this function were of special interest in achieving a user-friendly facility, and these areas were viewed as functioning almost as a hotel check-in.

The five areas listed above were divided into two zones, one dedicated to patient care and one that provided support. Programmatically these areas were roughly equal, and were grouped as follows:

Patient Care:
  Admission/discharge/patient service
  Patient Education and Treatment
Patient Support:
  Administration
  Food service/dining/housekeeping

Organization and interrelationship of the spaces was analyzed next. The committees developed patient and staff flow models which were tested against present practice and the NYU model. Process for each function was defined and established in writing by the committees. This method allowed each facet to be critically analyzed by administration, other disciplines, and for patient-focused care. It also allowed the architect to propose spatial relation concepts for critique. Pursuing this process within a committee structure was time-consuming, but it allowed each interest group or discipline to see and understand its relationships with others. Internal circulation also grew from this process, with a goal of simplicity and clarity for the patient. It became evident that a circular flow was functionally most efficient and also eliminated patient and care partner confusion. Circulation with respect to the remainder of the hospital also was studied. Connection to the hospital's main floor was considered essential for patients and care partners to easily access other hospital services. This analysis meant that the Cooperative Care Center's therapeutic floor had to be located one story above grade on the selected site to align it with the Rhode Island Hospital main floor level.

Specialized program items also were included for each area and recorded for future use; examples include a dedicated service elevator and a pneumatic tube system.

SITING

A Cooperative Care Center requires the same in-depth planning as do all hospital units. Of prime importance is the need to focus on the reality that the Cooperative Care Center is a true inpatient facility, with admission guidelines, patient care needs, and access to other hospital support systems given the same priority as in other inpatient facilities. However, these goals need to be attained in a different manner from a traditional hospital unit. The differences in these issues are sometimes subtle, but handling them properly is an important key to success. The following points are critical in making final architectural plans:

1. *Focus on patient and care partner convenience.* Most medical facilities are designed for the staff's convenience. This must be reversed if cooperative care is to be successful, as the care partner is the most essential individual in the patient's care.

2. *Provide a separate, distinct identity.* Difference from traditional hospital units should be emphasized so that administration, staff, and patient approach this undertaking with a new attitude and willingness to question standard approaches to patient care.

3. *Assure physical proximity to support facilities.* As in other inpatient facilities, patients must circulate to treatment and diagnostic areas. The knowledge that these facilities are close and available is especially important as reassurance to the patient and care partner.

4. *Design clear circulation routes.* The care partner will provide transportation services in the treatment process, so the circulation pattern must be clear and supported by user-friendly graphics.

5. *Separate from medically intensive activity.* Cooperative Care is a different, more hospitable, approach to care. This requires a change in atmosphere and attitude from the traditional inpatient unit. The architecture must support and encourage this difference.

6. *Control construction costs.* Cooperative care provides the opportunity to reduce operational costs on an ongoing basis. Initial construction costs also are greatly reduced compared to those of a typical inpatient unit. Siting of the facility can greatly affect initial construction cost. Least-cost alternatives must be tested against other identified goals.

7. *Design for people, not machines or process.* Sometimes overlooked in designing treatment spaces, the care partner and patient should be treated and housed as they would in a fine hotel.

8. *Ease access.* Arrival and departure must be user-friendly and patient-focused, utilizing elements from the hospitality industry to achieve this goal.

PLANNING INTERIOR DESIGN

The interior design process of a health care facility is much the same as in any other project. The phases are schematic design, design development, budget development, documentation, procurement assistance, project administration, and postevaluations. The design issues are typically: perceived image, design solutions, maintenance requirements, associated costs and, in this case, existing standards, as set by the Hasbro Children's Hospital project.

Innovative results come from carefully listening to those who understand the operational concept. In this case they resulted not only from the actual developers and end users, but also those who have created the Cooperative Care concept in another institution and those who have experience in providing service in both the health care and hospitality markets. It is important to define the market the client is seeking and determine how the design will strengthen their place in that market. It is important to portray the quality of service to be provided, in this case with comfort, convenience, clear direction and subtle diversion. It is imperative to provide the client with a project that creates a difference.

The design must be worked from the inside out. Researching a constantly changing market that will support your desired image while creating comfort and convenience is key to the process. Way-finding needs to be coordinated to reinforce one's sense of direction in a foreign environment. When you add stress to that environment it is important to add diversion through aesthetic detailing.

It is interesting to note the differences between the hospitality market and the health care market. Although both markets follow similar procedures for welcoming, receiving, checking in or admitting, assigning rooms, providing support services, and checking out or discharging, the nature of the service and the physical well-being of each market's guest is very different. There is also a perceived difference in the mind of the consumer about both of these markets.

In the hospitality market, hotel selection is usually an elective luxury that one chooses on the basis of location, convenience, and cost. In health care, however, a hospital is usually selected by one's referring physician based upon the nature of the procedure and the physician's privileges. Therefore, consumers traditionally have accepted much less in the health care environment than would ever be acceptable in a hospitality setting. Clearly that attitude is changing. There are now more choices in the health care delivery system, with more satellite facilities available to physicians and their patients. These facilities are competing for more of the market share. As a result, more of a hospitality attitude is emerging, as one of the ways in which individual institutions can maintain their competitive edges.

This project provided the opportunity to really meld some concepts and products from the hospitality industry with those of the health care industry. The hospitality market needed to be carefully scrutinized for its applicability in the health care environment. Typically, the hospitality market replaces finishes and furnishings every 3 to 5 years; the health care market traditionally replaces every 10 to 15 years. The hospitality interiors industry designs its products for the 3-to-5 year replacement cycle. Consequently, making the decision to use hospitality-designed products in the health care setting is a little difficult to justify, considering the extended length of service required.

Since maintenance is a very important issue in health care, all finishes and furnishings must be able to withstand a great deal of abuse in usage as well as in standard maintenance procedures. Bleach solutions are often used to clean and disinfect. Not all fibers and finishes will stand up to such harsh detergents and disinfectants. The result is the need to use health care-related finishes in a hospitality-related way.

The development of Senior Living Centers has encouraged many of the manufacturers of hospitality-related furnishings to take notice of the needs and demands of the end users in this market. Those companies that have done so have many more offerings than those entering the market fresh. From our point of view, furnishings that are upholstered or serve some function in physically supporting a patient are likely to be specified from one of these lines or from a traditional health care line.

The economic recession also has helped the interior designer and the health care industry to abandon a very predictable institutional look. Most manufacturers of interior finishes and furnishings have seen the once stronger markets in hospitality and corporate design dry up. With a boom in health care construction, all attention turned to retooling and redesigning to pick up a piece of this market share. To those of us who have been in the institutional market for a while, it became apparent that although the new styles and more intricately patterned finishes were a welcomed change, many of these companies had never dealt with the many complex needs of the health care end user. So with great caution, careful evaluation and much user review, we look beyond color choices and style selections to be sure our specifications are well suited for the end user, and that they have the ability to withstand 24 hours a day, 7 days a week's worth of tough use and abuse from a varied population. It is easy to deliver a project that looks good on dedication day and present a wonderful portfolio from the camera's eye, but you do not succeed in health care until the damage is done and the repairs are painless.

Postevaluations and final reviews are especially necessary on this project, since new trails have been blazed. It is important that new staff members are oriented to the design, that the concepts are understood, and that all systems in the design process are working as harmoniously as planned.

23

A HOTEL/HEALTH CARE ALLIANCE: THE PATIENT AS GUEST

Richard H. Kennedy and Theodore W. Kinkel

This chapter will discuss the planning of the Cooperative Care Center of Rhode Island from the perspective of providing an exceptional guest experience for patients, so that they will recommend the Cooperative Care Center of Rhode Island to others. It will demonstrate the benefits of a strategic alliance between the hospitality and health care industries, and will include examples of processes and techniques used to maximize the effectiveness of this alliance.

WHAT REALLY MATTERS

Other than achieving a favorable medical outcome, hospitals traditionally have given limited thought to what really matters to the patient.

Good medical care, a clean room, and a competent nurse have, in the past, defined quality to a significant degree. By the very nature of the cooperative care philosophy, which emphasizes empowering the patient to be more independent than dependent, health care managers are encouraged to have the customers define quality according to their own needs and values. Once this focus has been recognized and accepted by those responsible for planning and implementing a cooperative care unit, a dramatic, positive improvement in customer service and satisfaction can occur. For the Rhode Island/Women & Infant's Cooperative Care Center, this shift in orientation and focus is designated as Guest Services.

Cultivating the appropriate mindset to accept and implement the change in customer orientation is difficult. Managers trained in traditional health care delivery hold powerful paradigms regarding their concept of "guest service" in health care. Before it is possible to implement positive improvement in guest services, we need to recognize these paradigms and move through an *evolutionary* process in which we encounter, explore, and challenge both traditional and new guest service concepts.

Real change in the guest service focus resulted from an alliance with representatives from Marriott Health Care Services, who brought to our meetings their commitment to defining customer needs and exceeding their expectations. Their philosophy, values, guest service experience, and ongoing challenge of the way we viewed service contributed to the recognition of these traditional paradigms and the need for a constructive climate for change. We know that if we are to fulfill our commitment to continuous quality improvement and to patient-centered care, our current view of the world and past practices should not be obstacles. Without a fundamental determination to do more than permit a care partner to participate in the care of the patient and to provide a hotel-like room to stay in, the Cooperative Care philosophy will not be realized.

Benchmarking the best practices you can find in guest services is a good way to start the process of making this fundamental change. The hotel industry offers exceptional models for the delivery of services that matter to the guest. Their goals are similar to those of hospitals: to ensure an exceptional experience and build intent for the guests to positively recommend their hotel to others. Those most successful in the hospitality industry have solid and often fascinating research on customer preferences and priorities that guide their decisions. This ongoing willingness to ask the customer, analyze the data, and respond to what is learned is a salient lesson.

For example, Marriott conducted research that concluded that the five key drivers that have the greatest impact on overall guest satisfaction and intent to return are cleanliness, value, breakfast, friendliness, and check-in speed. Guest needs were identified to be: No anxiety or surprises, guest recognition (by name), no wasted time or effort, hospitable service, no handoffs from one employee to another to make decisions on behalf of the guest, and quick and efficient problem resolution.

With this knowledge, it was determined that if positive changes could be made in the "First Ten" minutes of a guest's stay beginning at registration, striking improvement in guest satisfaction could occur and Marriott could attain both customer service and competitive advantages. The "First Ten" check-in processes were redesigned around guest needs. This included ensuring each guest a warm greeting immediately upon arrival; personalized name recognition for repeat guests; personalized service with all administrative functions such as room assignment, method of payment, and availability of the room key completed prior to arrival; confirmation of room rate, room type, departure date, and method of payment; allowing the guest the ability to go directly to the room and bypass the front desk; and clean, comfortable guest rooms where everything is in working order.

Today, Marriott is implementing its new guest service concept in its hotels and inns as well as in the 1200 health care facilities with which it has management contracts for one or more departments. It has faced challenges similar to what health care executives may experience as we rethink and improve guest service activities. These challenges include eliminating traditional departmental and cultural barriers; creating broadly defined, multifunctional jobs; automating administrative functions; eliminating all non-value-added functions; and implementing sensitive guest satisfaction measurement tools. *The Journal of Healthcare Quality* offers many suggestions of how to gather these data (Quinn, 1992). After satisfaction results are analyzed, the focus should return to the patient and care partner through the continuous improvement cycle.

The starting point for our paradigm shift is the guest, who was previously referred to as the patient. The use of this new word to describe the focus of our effort serves as a constant reminder to the service team that customer service needs to take on an unconventional and possibly new definition in health care. Simply stated, the connotation for "guest" is service and hospitality. We perceive the feelings of caring and warmth generated when we are a guest in someone's home or a service-rich hotel, or when dining out. Why should those undergoing medical care and their care partners not experience similar emotions and positive perceptions when they are guests in the hospital?

The philosophy of Cooperative Care encourages patients to play an active role in decisions regarding their own medical care, self-management, and relative independence. The care partner is given shared responsibilities for the administration of medications, for ensuring that the patient gets to scheduled appointments, and that the patient's comfort needs are met. To achieve this level of autonomy, structure and resources must be provided that permit the patient and care partner an unusual amount of independence through empowerment. Systems need to be operational that provide for needed care partner and patient training; make communication with their caregivers convenient and accessible at all times; and enable them to feel that they have a far greater level of control than is normally experienced in a hospital.

The Cooperative Care employee must be empowered to serve the patient and the care partner. This requires a redefinition of authority and responsibility that harnesses workers to quality promotion (Donabedian, 1993). The goal must be that each employee will accept responsibility for finding the answer to a question posed by a patient or care partner and for meeting that need.

Future health care services, from the hospitality industry's perspective, should be comprised of service-rich health care organizations characterized by multiskilled hourly associates (employees) working across traditional departmental lines; ease of customer service access; a vibrant service culture focused on exceeding the expectations of the guest; hotel service training; all processes and procedures designed to ensure a hassle-free guest experience; a manager designated to champion guest services; and associate synergy developed through acceptance and belief in a common purpose and mission. Supporting these will be hotel systems and integrated computer technology that will enable the associate to produce a service-rich environment and achieve exceptional guest satisfaction outcomes.

However, before genuine guest service can be achieved, the existing health care management mindset needs to shift. Hospital administrators, outside vendors acting as partners, caregivers, and department heads must blend their skills, ideas, and creative talents to design an organization, an operating system, and a physical plant that will enable the associates to deliver a customer-focused product and service. This synergy catalyzes, unifies, and unleashes the greatest powers within people and creates new alternatives (Covey, 1989). Developing buy-in and commitment is critical to future success. For the Cooperative Care Center of Rhode Island, quality improvement processes and large group meeting techniques have been used in developing a vigorous customer focus. Our story, while not unique, may shed some light on how a vendor-partner relationship can develop and thrive, and how the paradigms relative to exceptional guest service may be changed.

The following is a summary of key outcomes and observations of a chronological sequence of retreats held by Rhode Island Hospital, Women and Infant's Hospital, and Marriott Health Care Service. The word "retreat" is significant as it indicates that the series of meetings was important enough to hold away from the hospital property to insure an atmosphere free of interruption, day-to-day management activities, and appropriate for creative thinking.

STRATEGIC REVIEW RETREAT

The first meeting of the hospitals and Marriott was scheduled as a two-day retreat with senior leadership and executives to share and build consensus around group norms. The following questions and concerns were explored, presented, and discussed:

- If this meeting is to be successful for me, it must . . . ?
- My concerns about this undertaking are . . . ?
- How will we communicate to those who are not here, but are interested in what we are doing?
- Share detailed strategic plans of all prospective partners to thoroughly understand the direction and resources of each business unit.
- Build *trust* in personal and business relationships with senior executives, so vital to developing a synergistic effort.
- Share Marriott research on the key drivers of guest satisfaction that have the greatest impact on the overall quality service satisfaction and intent to return. [The intent of this segment of the retreat was to hear hard research data regarding *what is important to the hotel guest* and to begin the evolution of a *health care guest paradigm shift.*]
- Explore what is possible with the new relationship and what is the value to each partner. [This was a particularly meaningful segment as can be seen from the "out of the box" ideas that were generated.]

What is Possible?

- Develop a common vision for medical and non-medical care.
- Maximize guest satisfaction.
- Develop a strong patient preference for cooperative care.

- Explore what we can provide together that adds value to the guest experience.
- Significantly improve the admission procedures to include speed, friendliness, courtesy, and guest satisfaction.
- Establish a laboratory for multiskilled staff.
- Under one guest services champion, manage all hotel and hospitality functions.
- Serve as a laboratory to pilot ideas, test and refine guest service processes, and if successful, share and implement beyond the Cooperative Care Center.

What is the Value to Rhode Island Hospital and Women and Infants Hospital?

- Become a low-cost producer.
- Maximize the perception and reality of quality.
- Focus on patient service needs.
- Stimulate management to look at guest services from a customer's perspective.
- Enhance the effectiveness of the hospital management by working together on a significant campus project.
- Build our collective skills in quality improvement.

What is the Value to Marriott?

- Provide a fast track on revolutionary concepts.
- Achieve additional tools to be a low cost/high quality provider.
- Bring together Marriott Hotels, Resorts, Suites, and Marriott Health Care Services systems and technology.
- Offer a stimulus to look at things differently.
- Develop a profile for future success to include skills in developing a joint venture and a working research laboratory.
- Serve as a training site for multiskilled managers and associates.
- Develop a consolidated guest service/hospitality product line.

This meeting turned out to be the foundation for the beginning of a highly successful vendor alliance. Our collective success would not have been achieved had the executive team not cleared their calendars and committed themselves to fully capitalize on the potential of this new business relationship.

"FOCUS ON THE GUEST" RETREAT

The focus of this two-day second retreat was to answer a simple yet complex question:

How should/will the guest experience/process in the Cooperative Care Center be different from a standard hospital experience/process? Who is the customer and what contributes positively to the overall guest experience?

The meeting was facilitated by an executive trained in quality improvement and interactive meeting techniques. This assured that a highly spirited and creative meeting achieved a high degree of focus and tangible/actionable outcomes. Participation in the retreat was expanded to include physician representation, to secure a more complete perspective and diversity of viewpoints.

Who is the Customer?

Exploration of this question expanded the normal definition of the customer as the patient to include the care partner—really emphasized for the first time—the physician, the nurse, third-party payors, employer, family/children, visitors, and employees, as well as the patient. This highly stimulating and productive activity focussed on the preopening phases of cooperative care, guest preadmission, guest admission, guest stay/care, and guest discharge. The process resulted in more than ten typewritten pages of suggestions that were thought to produce a composite positive guest experience in the new Cooperative Care Center. These suggestions have formed the basis for future decisions relative to guest room amenities, communication technology and software, role delineation, staffing and management organization, and, most importantly, the mission statement of the Cooperative Care Center.

COOPERATIVE CARE PLANNING RETREAT

The third retreat expanded the number of participants from an average of 10 to more than 40 managers and department heads from Rhode Island Hospital, Women and Infants Hospital, and Marriott Health Care Services. Again the meeting was held away from the hospitals to maximize the synergy for those participating. The objectives of this retreat were to:

1. Develop a common database and ownership of the vision of the Cooperative Care Center among all participants by having them share and contribute in a large group interactive meeting process.

2. Establish a guest service vision and mission statement for the Cooperative Care Center.

3. Initiate an organization structure to manage the process through successful implementation.

Two professional meeting facilitators representing Rhode Island Hospital and Marriott Health Care Services developed the two-day meeting design and facilitated the meeting. Participants were assigned to discussion tables in a maximum mix manner. The purpose was to insure that the maximum diversity of personnel was represented in each discussion group and to develop a working relationship between hospital and Marriott representatives who were unfamiliar with each other.

Participants established and shared their perspective for desired meeting outcomes and ground rules for participation. These exercises helped to put people at ease and add clarity and focus to the retreat.

Desired Outcomes

The group decided to jointly develop a vision/mission for the Cooperative Care Center that would drive an implementation plan built on creative thinking and consensus. The commitment was made to continually refocus our thinking on the patient's needs and on those of the care partner and family.

Participants brainstormed the question: "What will it take to ensure that the Cooperative Care Center is wildly successful, as seen by the following groups: patient, care partner and family, staff, physician, payor/employer, owners, and community-at-large?" Presentations were made and discussion followed in order to achieve the perspective of this expanded group of managers. Following this activity, the following futuristic scenario, "A Vision for the Future—The Guest's Perspective" was read.

> Visiting her physician, Mrs. Howard and her husband have just learned that she will require hospitalization for surgery. After explaining the procedure and the anticipated recovery, her doctor introduces Mr. and Mrs. Howard to the Cooperative Care Center, a new kind of hospital in Providence. Following a suggestion by their physician, the couple read and discuss a small pamphlet which clearly outlines the benefits of this new health care environment.
>
> After expressing some interest in exploring further the nontraditional

hospital option, they are comfortably seated in front of an "interactive, color, computer monitor" by the physician's receptionist. Within a few moments, the receptionist has made a telephone connection and Mr. and Mrs. Howard are introduced "visually" and through voice transmission to Betsey, a Guest Service Associate of the Cooperative Care Center.

Their first experience is enhanced by human elements, a trained staff member, a cheerful greeting, an attractive professional appearance, and an expression of real interest in service. The Howards are impressed by the personal warmth conveyed via the state-of-the-art technology that makes this all possible. Betsey, picking up on visual cues as well as the conversational exchange, determines that the Cooperative Care Center is a viable and realistic hospitalization alternative for the Howards.

To provide a thorough introduction, the receptionist plays a short introductory video for the Howards. The video explains the service-rich, caring, warm environment, the role of the care partner, and puts them at ease by sharing the breadth of medical expertise available on the Rhode Island and Women and Infant's Hospital Campus. Mr. Howard exclaims: 'This is nothing like I expected! I can stay with my wife in the privacy of a modern hotel, assist her through her illness and recovery, and even go to work.'

The decision by Mr. and Mrs Howard to accept the Cooperative Care hospitalization option is made following a brief discussion of its many advantages and the opportunity to ask any questions regarding this concept of care. Within an additional 5 minutes, Betsey, the Guest Service Associate, receives and simultaneously inputs all necessary admitting and guest information into the management information system. On the color video display, the Howards are able to see their admitting information once input, and are able to verify the accuracy of all entries. Betsey inquires and receives permission to take a quick snapshot picture of the Howards to assist her and the staff in recognizing them upon their arrival. With the click of a computer mouse, the video display of the Howards is turned into a low resolution photograph. Within a few moments, Betsey has all that is needed, and the date and time of admission is confirmed.

With the Howards' stay now a week away, they receive in the mail a personalized letter of welcome from Betsey, along with a packet outlining the available guest services. Comfortable with their knowledge of the things to pack and the positive experience to anticipate, their preparation for the hospital visit is relaxing rather than anxiety-filled.

The drive to Providence is filled with conversation on what the experience will be like. Mr. Howard expresses some concern and a little apprehension. Mrs. Howard humorously wonders, "Who is going in the hospital, my husband or me?" Leaving the interstate, they see large signs directing them to the covered drive and entrance to the Cooperative Care Center. Mr. Howard pulls the car under the protective canopy and is immediately greeted by a uniformed Cooperative Care Center Associate.

Mr. and Mrs. Howard are surprised to be greeted by name, but then remember that Betsey previously had taken a photograph of them during the admission procedure performed at the doctor's office.

Assistance is provided to load their luggage on a hotel luggage cart and Mr. Howard decides to self-park in the secured and private patient parking lot. Upon entering, he notes the privacy gate insuring convenient and private guest parking. He thinks to himself, "Parking could not be simpler." By the time Mr. Howard rides the elevator to the reception area of the Cooperative Care Center, his wife has already been escorted to the lobby by Betsey, and is waiting for him. Upon arrival, Betsey greets Mr. Howard and they proceed directly to their hotel-like room.

Walking off the elevator, they see a large-scale, easy-to-read, colorful map of the Care Center and campus. Conveniently, smaller maps are folded and available for their use at any time. As they proceed, Betsey familiarizes the Howards with various guest facilities and services—little things, like how to open the room door with their disposable room key which enhances guest security. After helping Mr. and Mrs. Howard with their luggage, Betsey begins a well planned orientation to the guest room. In addition to ensuring their comfort, the orientation is designed to maximize their safety. Starting with the bedside and desk telephones, they recognize that this is not your typical hospital. Both direct dial phones are equipped with a hands-free speaker phone; large, easy-to-read-and-use buttons; and a port for a computer modem. The Howards learn that the phones have been configured to allow both of them to listen and speak with their physician. Mr. Howard notices the desk, work light, and even a modem connection if he chooses to do a little work and communicate to his office. He exclaims, "What a great idea! It looks like you've thought of everything. I can be with my wife and not have to worry about the work piling up with access to this modern communication system." Betsy reminds him of the facsimile service available in the reception area.

Continuing with their orientation, they are taught to operate the remote control television with access to all major networks, basic cable, and sports. Quickly, Betsy demonstrates how to access the scheduling channel, which displays Mrs. Howard's personal appointments with physicians; and the guest service channel which features the menu for each meal, the support groups and classes that are meeting, as well as the hours of service and locations of such services as the mail, barber and beauty, flowers, and the library. Like any modern hotel, they have access to pay-per-view with the latest movies. They also have access to a free library of health care videos designed to educate and answer questions.

Betsey then speaks of the most important channel that is required watching for all first-time and repeat guests of the Cooperative Care Center. *'Welcome and Familiarization'* is shown every half-hour. All guests, patient and care partner, watch this video designed to welcome, familiarize, and to ensure a safe, pleasant, and medically responsible experience.

After providing detailed information on the hotel services, it reviews safety procedures, such as what to do in case of a medical emergency, fire, or fall. The responsibilities of the care partner are explained in a simple, step-by-step procedure. At the end of the video, the care partner and patient are directed to open the guest services booklet, retrieve the orientation review form, read, sign, and return it to the reception desk during the first day of their stay. Documentation of the self-administered orientation is monitored and discussed at their first meeting with their nurse clinician.

With a quick demonstration, they are shown how to use the television screen to answer questions after viewing video instructional tapes. This allows the Howards and their nurse clinician to confirm their level of understanding and comprehension of any instructional videos regarding treatment plans. The last service discussed on their room television is the billing update. Services which are available but not customarily covered by the Howards' medical insurance may be purchased. Additional amenities such as room service, flowers, magazines, long distance telephone service, movies and pay-per-view events may be charged to their account by simply presenting their personal Cooperative Care charge card. The charge card indicates that the Howards have established an account and wish to authorize billing for additional services available at the Cooperative Care Center.

The orientation to their hotel-style room continues as Betsey points out the medically necessary needle box and covered receptacle for wound dressings, located in the lavatory. They are reminded of the health and safety reasons for these devices and the proper means to use them. The grab bars in the tub and the handicap-equipped devices are pointed out. Mrs. Howard is pleased to see the instant hot water, coffee cups, tea, and coffee. Other conveniences, such as the wall-mounted hair dryer, ironing board and iron, room safe, and mini-refrigerator, are all designed to make their stay truly delightful and hassle-free. Somebody seems to have thought of everything.

Completing their orientation, Betsey and the Howards sit down at the round conference style table located in each room. Equipped with four chairs, it looks like a great place to play some games with their grandchildren or visit with friends. But today, Betsey uses it to complete the admission process, something she started weeks ago with the Howards when they were in the physician's office. Thus, only one person conducted the entire admissions process, welcome, orientation, provided personal assistance, and answered questions for the Howards.

At the end of the process, Mrs. Howard is given a small, almost pocket-sized, cellular telephone for use inside the Cooperative Care Center. Betsey explains that from time to time, she may receive a call on the phone to remind her of scheduled appointments or changes in schedule, or perhaps from her physician or even her husband. The cellular telephone works on the same number as the Howards' Cooperative Care Center hotel room. She is shown how to use it and how to store it at night so that the batteries are able to recharge.

Mr. Howard is provided with a wide-area-display beeper that will be used by the staff in case they need to call him while in the building or anywhere in the Providence or Boston area. It is explained to the Howards that, like them, the telephone and beeper are a matched set. Clearly inscribed on each one are instructions and numbers to allow them to directly call the other.

Comforted by the courtesy and warmth of the CCC staff, the Howards rest for a while and then make their way to the dining room for their first meal. Immediately upon entering the dining room, they are impressed by the crisp and attractive atmosphere. They receive a warm and genuine greeting from an attractively uniformed guest service associate who introduces herself and inquires if she may review meal service with them.

Upon walking through the service area, they see attractive displays of food presented for self- and assisted service. They note the variety and the clear point-of-service signs that identify the menu of the day. Mrs. Howard has an appointment made with the dietitian to review the diet she has ordered and they are then escorted through the cafeteria line to select their meal.

The intent of this scenario was to share another viewpoint of what was possible and to further expand the creative thinking and remove existing paradigms. Whether the vision was accepted or not, the process was valuable, as it opened up and identified further opportunities and acceptance for improvement in guest services.

This vision and the exercises during the retreat led to the development of the mission statement for the Cooperative Care Center:

> The mission of the Cooperative Care Center is to provide quality health care services in a hospital setting, where teams of health care professionals join patients and their care partners to treat and manage the patient's illness, with an emphasis on patient education and autonomy. This setting combines the comforts of home with the amenities of a hotel and the security of a hospital. This innovative environment sets a new standard for value in the delivery of health care.

Formation of a series of teams was recommended to provide the future leadership and organizational structure for the implementation and operation of the Cooperative Care Center. Team structure was designed to reflect the philosophy of the partner institutions. All of the business partners have worked to develop a strategic alliance built on mutual respect and trust and wins for all those involved. We understand that if we unselfishly pool our efforts, and concentrate on making the guests' stay at the Cooperative Care Center the most favorable experience possible, all of our organizations will benefit. Each person who has been actively involved in the alliance has grown personally and professionally. We feel that we are better prepared to handle the future challenges of health care reform, have learned the value of continuous improvement activities, and have witnessed and shared in the synergy and positive energy developed from a highly effective team.

PLANNING FOR IMPLEMENTATION

Kenneth Weiner, Donald E. Schildkamp, and
Daniel D. Hanlon

THE ACTIVATION MANAGEMENT PLAN

The activation management plan is a one-year plan to guide the preparation for and opening of the Cooperative Care Center. As such, it describes an organizational structure that provides a working framework for communications and lines of responsibility. It also serves as a conduit for task identification and problem resolution among the teams.

OPERATIONS PLANNING

The objective of the management plan is to provide a framework to guide and coordinate the many activities required to successfully prepare, open, and operate the Cooperative Care Center consistent with its mission. Values were heavily emphasized in the planning of this document. The values included were:

1. Processes will be designed and implemented from the patient's point of view.

2. Every effort will be made to support the care partners and encourage their participation in the care of the patient.

3. Care and patient service will be patient-focused.

4. Employees will be multiskilled, flexible and empowered.

5. The overall atmosphere and culture will be warm, friendly, and inviting.

6. The interests of all stakeholders will be actively sought and considered.

7. Communication and education will be consistently encouraged.

The general strategy that was used to design this process was first to identify and develop the processes and procedures needed to run the facility; second, to develop descriptions of the tasks, jobs, and positions required to carry out the processes and procedures; and third, to develop budgets.

The various teams were charged with developing processes for the tasks that fell under their respective rubrics, to develop descriptions of jobs and staffing needs, and to look at the financial impact of what they are doing. This was an iterative process. Each department was given an opportunity to re-evaluate and improve departmental work processes.

The approach taken for the design and implementation of policies and procedures was to employ eight action teams and a coordination team to which they report. Action teams are variously composed of representatives from each department that is impacted by the tasks undertaken by that team. The cross-departmental mix of the Action Teams membership ensures effective communication across functional lines.

Coordination Team

The objective of the coordination team is to provide the overall direction and coordination needed to successfully bring the facility online as well as to facilitate interteam communication. That team will be responsible for successful activation of the Cooperative Care Center. Its standing members include the Executive Director, Medical Director, clinical director of the new center, Senior Management Engineer, Human Resource Generalist, and Chairmen of other committees. The Coordination team's tasks are to:

1. Define global, temporal, and procedural standards;
2. Establish overall priorities;

3. Define reporting procedures;
4. Define documentation standards;
5. Establish Action Teams and appoint team leaders;
6. Organize and hold initial chairperson tasking meeting;
7. Plan guidelines:
8. Propose initial Action Team name and objectives;
9. Identify and allocate resources;
10. Develop operating budget;
11. Develop staffing estimates;
12. Compile overall assumptions and constraints.

Action Teams

There are eight Action Teams, each of them comprised of representatives of all participating agencies. Tasks and goals are being accomplished in accordance with each team's own schedule and procedures.
This, in turn, will support the overall project milestone schedule. Formation and dissolution of subcommittees, ad hoc task forces, etc., is encouraged at the discretion of the action teams.

Major products of the action teams are: process identification and
development, staffing estimates, task descriptions, training, and education. The teams are organized around major process areas which cut
across functional lines. Team construction reflects the basic structure
and organizational culture of the institution in which the project is to
be implemented. The approach taken by the Cooperative Care Center
of Rhode Island would not necessarily work in other settings.

Project management is required to ensure that all tasks are accounted for, scheduled, and completed in a timely manner. At the
heart of this plan is the concept of a collaborative and highly commu-
nicative environment, where every employee feels comfortable enough
to rise to the challenge of providing more effective care to patients
while consuming fewer resources. Staff at all levels of the organization
will be encouraged at all times to look at the way things are done and
at how they could do them better. Corporate culture and incentives designed into the processes will foster this desired perspective.

BUDGET PLANNING

The initial intention in budget planning was that the staffing requirements developed by the teams would drive the salary portion of the

budget. However, because the entire planning process was slightly behind the budgetary cycle, a tentative budget was established offline with input from department directors and other executive personnel.

STAFFING REQUIREMENTS

There are two significant differences in staffing patterns between Cooperative Care and nursing units in the main hospital. The first is the decreased number of nurses which results from the use of care partners. Nursing ratios in the Cooperative Care Center are expected to be similar to NYU's unit, namely 1:13–15, compared with 1:5 on an average medical/surgical floor in the main hospital. This should result in a savings of up to 30% in staff salary expenses.

The second unique feature is the focus on hospitality, with resultant introduction of guest service associates whose jobs will be to provide hotel-like services and amenities.

COLLABORATIVE ATMOSPHERE

The process we have chosen is only one of many possible approaches an organization can take. In an environment where the culture does not support teamwork or collaboration, it would be difficult to structure and implement a process that involves working in teams. Some would argue that teams are an unnecessary drain on organizational manpower. It could be argued that decisions are made and acted upon more quickly with fewer people and fewer meetings. This may be true; however, the effectiveness of those decisions, actions, and outcomes will always be greater if made collectively in a healthy, well-performing, diversified team. People respond better to changes when they have a voice in the decisions that affect them. In this environment, experience has demonstrated that people working in teams do in fact yield better results than do the combined efforts of people working individually.

TEAM BUILDING AND TEAM LEADERSHIP TRAINING

Leading a cross-functional team requires different skills than managing a function. The Human Resource Department at RIH developed a Team Leadership training session specifically for this project. The training consisted of components on meeting effectiveness, learning/decisionmaking styles, understanding group process, and elements of successful teams. Just as there are different skills required to lead a team, there are also different behaviors required for functioning as part of a team.

Four things are important when selecting team leadership and membership and launching the teams. They are:

1. Establish criteria for selection of team leaders and team members. There are certain qualities or characteristics that are conducive to team work and some that get in the way;
2. Define the scope, boundaries, and resource availability to the team leader; allow some room for negotiation;
3. Make sure the team knows its purpose or reason for being, as well as the expectations; and
4. Provide training to the team leader and team members.

The dynamics of the group can have a significant impact on the outcome of the project. A dysfunctional team may not reach its objectives, and can create unresolved conflict that may be unhealthy for employee morale and relations as well as potentially compromising the overall project.

ADVANTAGES AND DISADVANTAGES OF CROSS-FUNCTIONAL TEAM STRUCTURE

Having departmental representation and involvement in decisionmaking creates a sense of ownership and can reduce, but not eliminate, resistance to change. It also greatly increases communications between and among departments and increases awareness, understanding, and appreciation for how each function fits within the organization. Having different perspectives, experience, and expertise represented will produce a product which is much different than one produced by a team comprised of people who are involved with one single function.

Cross-functional team structure requires skilled team leadership. This can be a disadvantage if there is a shortage of such leadership in an organization. For example, a big disadvantage of this approach is that it can be difficult to assemble all members of the team for regular meetings. It also requires more time away from normal job functions.

DECISIONS BY CONSENSUS

In large groups such as gathered for the retreat, it can be very difficult, if not impossible, to arrive at decisions with which everyone agrees. This can be difficult even in smaller groups. The problem is that each person may have a different need, expectation, or level of knowledge and experience that supports his or her position.

Making decisions by consensus can help a team perform at a level that exceeds individual performance. In order for a group of people to agree to accept and support a decision, there must be discussion, negotiation, and sometimes conflict. Difficult as this may be at times, it is important that the people working in groups be able to freely state their concerns, be respected for doing so, and be respectful of others as well.

How these elements are handled in the team will determine the value of the decision and the health of the team. Decision making by majority vote differs in that the team may not address all the important considerations or consequences before a vote is cast. It is a quick, nonconfrontational method that doesn't explore rationale and consequences. This type of decision making or resolution can lead to individual competitiveness within the team and a "win" or "lose" attitude. The essence of team performance lies not only with the team leader, but also in the relationships of those represented and participating on the team.

INTERTEAM COMMUNICATION

One significant advantage of working with cross-functional teams is an increased amount of communication. With a project of this scope, it is imperative that no one individual, group, or department operate without understanding what is going on in other work groups and departments. There must be cross-communication between departmental lines to eliminate redundant efforts, ensure nothing gets forgotten, and ensure understanding throughout the project. In our project, the charge of the team leader was to create a team that had representation from areas impacted by the design of the team; anyone else who would be involved in any process assigned to the team, and any one else who might add value to the design.

Since cooperative care by its very nature creates a collaborative environment, the collaborative group and team process we used for planning for implementation was a natural fit with this philosophy.

25

NURSING ISSUES AND PERSPECTIVES

Chrysanthe C. Stamoulis

PERSONAL REFLECTIONS

My introduction to the cooperative care concept, as defined by the NYU model, happened in 1987. I was then Director of Surgical Nursing. The Director of Medical Nursing and I went to New York that year to see if the model was applicable to our patient population and, more important, whether the concept was one that provided quality patient care in a cost-effective manner. Our trip to NYU really made us believe that there was something innovative and special going on in their hospital. It was obviously well set-up from a facility point of view. The building promoted patient and family independence. The therapeutic floor, the common rooms, and the separate "hotel like" patient and family quarters were a major paradigm shift for me. I remember commenting, "I don't think it will play in Providence!"

I did, however, have the impression that patients and their families appeared to be satisfied with the kind of care they were receiving, and that they understood planned procedures and expected outcomes.

There was a shared feeling that the family was central to all that the staff were doing at the hospital.

It also was interesting to watch the nurses in action and observe how they provided care and interacted with other members of the health care team. They really seemed to be quite satisfied with the care they provided, and found it very challenging and rewarding to practice the "essence of nursing." We spent a great deal of time with the nursing leaders discussing staffing, patient selection, physician collaboration and patient education.

When we came back from that first visit, we were excited by the idea and the model. However, it appeared to us that many of the patients in our hospital were more acutely ill than were the cooperative care patients at NYU. A number of our oncology patients already were being treated in an ambulatory setting in the George Day Hospital. Furthermore, we questioned some of the staffing assumptions, given our patient population and lack of Intensive Care Unit beds. Although a 719–bed hospital, RIH traditionally has had very few intensive care beds relative to other hospitals of its size. Even today, it has only 32 intensive care beds.

As a result of this anomaly, many patients who in other settings would be placed in intensive care beds are placed in four-bedded semiprivate rooms, our most prevalent type of accommodation, where they can be matched with lower acuity patients who help to keep an eye on them. Essentially, while we thought the NYU model was cost-effective and innovative, administration also was not sure if it would "play in Providence," and put it on the shelf until later, when it finally was brought forward once again by Bruce Komiske.

On my second visit to NYU, it was clear to me that patients were more acutely ill than they had seemed on my first visit. In conversation with the staff, they validated that they were experiencing a major shift to outpatient care. Nonetheless, the concept still worked, and the patients and families were satisfied with the services they were receiving. Equally important, the physicians, nursing staff, and other members of the team seemed to be able to provide quality patient care and experience job satisfaction. By the end of that visit, I was sold on Cooperative Care. I realized that the model was a viable concept that needed to be marketed to our patient care staff and patients.

I began a dialogue with our nurses, mainly to see how they would respond to the Cooperative Care concept. At first I think they thought it was absolutely crazy. It just didn't seem to make sense at all. How could I suggest that putting a hospital-level patient, with a care partner—whatever that meant—in a room and letting them lock the door was providing quality patient care? And how could a nurse provide care if she or he could not constantly observe and evaluate the patient? Many physicians believed that few families would be willing to help provide care in the hospital. Three nurses for 74 patients on the night shift . . . and so it went!

We discussed physician satisfaction with Cooperative Care and used many of our observations from NYU. For example, one criterion of physician satisfaction was that they could visit with and examine their patients in the therapeutic area and not have to go from room to room all over the hospital.

With the assistance of a Brown University medical student, we surveyed our patients to learn whether they would be willing to be admitted to a Cooperative Care facility if it were available. We also interviewed their families to see if they would be willing to provide daily assistance and stay with the patient in a homelike atmosphere. The consensus was that patients and their partners would consider the Cooperative Care Center, as there was added value in having the family learn more about how to take care of their loved ones, and patients were able to have care provided in a very dignified and humane way.

I had the attention of the nurses when I discussed the other aspects of the model. Staff were pleased to hear that most of what they considered to be nondirect patient care functions would be done by other workers. As a group, we began to look at innovative ways to deliver patient care, care that was the essence of nursing. We talked about teaching patients and their partners about wellness and the prevention of disease, and about coping with chronic illnesses and death. We discussed adding value to all our interactions with our patients and their families.

At first the nurses responded that it made sense. They did not have to make patients' beds, and there was no need for them to spend a lot of time cleaning up a patient's environment when they would rather just sit down with a patient and provide support and reassurance about a recent diagnosis or other problem. Nurses become frustrated when emotional or educational needs are neglected while they are caught up in the tasks of documentation and non-nursing functions.

In talking to the nurses about all the rewards and challenges of the Cooperative Care model, we also discussed the cost/benefit of care partners.

During this period of time, when we were trying to sell the Cooperative Care concept, I, unfortunately, had to go through two family members' illnesses and deaths from cancer. In one instance it was very evident that a Cooperative Care setting would have been beneficial. That one was my brother-in-law. His wife and family were in attendance all the time. His wife bathed him, fed him, watched his intravenous line, and did his colostomy care. He required a minimal amount of highly specialized nursing care during many of his hospitalizations. Care was given by many different nurses with many of the procedures done differently. It was hard for my sister-in-law to understand why they could not do his colostomy care the same way, and, more important, in the way he used to do it at home.

What also was difficult and frustrating was that when my brother-in-law came into the hospital because of an exacerbation of his symptoms over the five years of his illness, he would be put back into a dependent state. He was undressed and put on bed rest; his medications would be given according to hospital schedules; and his meals were on a different schedule and provided little variety to stimulate good nutrition. It would take him a long time after each hospitalization to get his strength back and start walking again. Much cajoling was required to encourage him to be independent, and to get back on a more reasonable schedule with meals and medications.

The idea of Cooperative Care absolutely makes so much sense, especially when we care for patients with chronic illness, and particularly a terminal illness, such as cancer. The outcome is probably better when a patient is treated in a Cooperative Care setting. When patients remain in control, they maintain their strength and their dignity, and have more hope about their future. Furthermore, I think their families and partners do not experience the powerlessness that so often develops in the routine hospital care setting. When patients come into the hospital we do everything we can to fit their needs and wants, as well as those of their family, into the hospital schedule. We rarely stop and take the opportunity to find out how the hospital fits into the patient's family.

WORK RESTRUCTURING

The staffing plan for Cooperative Care will significantly reduce the costs of health care delivery. However, costs also can be contained by using appropriate technology and work simplification. Every effort will be made prior to opening the new unit to redesign workflow in a manner that eliminates all functions that create frustration and do not add value to patient care or family education.

Multidisciplinary focus groups have been formed to review all patient care, clerical, environmental and service processes. The goal is to develop a model for patient care delivery that responds to health care reform, positions the hospital favorably in competitive markets, promotes collaboration with all members of the health care team, and does so while adhering to the Cooperative Care philosophy.

The Cooperative Care Center of Rhode Island will utilize nurses in a different manner than they are used at NYU. For example, after one of the earlier trips to NYU, we made the decision to combine the clinical and educational roles into one level of Master's-prepared educator/clinician. In observing the NYU nursing staff, which is divided into two teams, "clinical nurses" and "nurse-educators," it appeared that this model increased patient encounters and tended to isolate functions.

Over the years, clinical educators have demonstrated their ability to integrate educational expertise into a very patient-centered approach to caregiving. These individuals have a base in patient education, a global perspective on health care, exceptional critical thinking ability, and expert physical assessment and management skills. We believe that a model that combines these roles into one position will be more cost-effective and should increase patient satisfaction by providing continuity of care. Furthermore, it is our strong belief that nurse experts, unless they actually do provide care, cannot and do not maintain this expertise.

Each educator/clinician will have an associate technician assigned as a partner. The nurse will hire, evaluate and, if necessary, terminate the associate. We propose this model in an effort to streamline bureaucracy and management while promoting accountability and staff nurse empowerment. The technician's position will allow us to enrich current jobs and to provide employees a greater diversity of role, competency, and authority. The multiskilled technicians will be trained to provide venipunctures, phlebotomies, EKGs, and other designated technical tasks. Teamwork, collaboration, and communication will be of paramount concern.

COLLABORATIVE PRACTICE

As we move closer to the opening of the Cooperative Care Center of Rhode Island, it is imperative that we plan team building activities for the core staff. There also is a need for an initiative to address physician and nurse collaboration. NYU's success can be attributed to the outstanding partnership of physicians and nurses. The history of RIH and WIH is such that the culture has not always fostered these relationships in the past. In an effort to get the project off on the right track, both Medical and Nursing Directors will be appointed by the same search committee. Significant weight will be given to their ability to work collaboratively and successfully as partners. This is key to the success of this project!

Our nursing colleagues at NYU have been very supportive, pointing out the pitfalls over the years. They maintain that once physicians use the services they are sold on the concept. Patients not only request Cooperative Care, but sometimes refuse to be admitted if there is no Cooperative Care bed available. Other professionals for the most part, had few problems, as their services were delivered in much the same way regardless of the setting.

STAFF NURSE ACCEPTANCE

The NYU staff mentioned that the greatest problem was with staff nurse acceptance. Staff nurses found it very difficult. They were used to being in charge. Nurses are accustomed to having patients dependent upon them. How could a patient and family member be allowed to walk up to their room and hide behind a locked door for the afternoon? No matter how much we may talk about this and try to prepare for this role change, it will be difficult, because it strikes at the essence of the caretaking role that nurses have provided for years. Patients are dependent upon us, and there has been almost a codependency around that role. Nurses have a difficult time letting go. The literature is replete with how nurses assume maternal roles and often treat patients almost like children. They care for them and see them in a dependent role.

As patients begin to pay more out of pocket for their health care, they will be demanding more. Patients want to have and are willing to pay for, the ambiance of home while being treated by a highly professional staff. Third-party payors will be looking for hospitals and networks in which innovative methods are being used to reduce length of stay, provide quality services cost-effectively, and provide health education to effect outcomes and to reduce readmissions. We are sure that many of the services provided by Cooperative Care would meet and often exceed their expectations.

ACKNOWLEDGEMENTS

With special thanks to Jane Wernig, Director of Nursing Professional Development at Rhode Island Hospital, who was responsible for the work restructuring program.

26

MEDICAL STAFF ISSUES

Richard A. Browning, Christopher J. Morin, and
Steven M. Sepe

The NYU Cooperative Care Center certainly was something new to
the Rhode Island Hospital medical staff who were first introduced to it
in 1988. There was some interest at that time but no consensus that
this was more than a novelty. There also was considerable confusion
over what the concept really was. Since, except for Intensive Care
Units, inpatient hospital facilities have not really changed over the
last 50 years, it was difficult to visualize how this new hospital unit
would work.

The first hurdle for physician staff support was to break down some
of the rules about how an inpatient service had to operate. After several presentations, there still was considerable confusion over what exactly this new concept and facility was. Misperceptions were frequent.
Staff physicians thought it was a step-down unit, a nursing home, a
hotel, a day hospital, or just about everything else except an inpatient
unit. Without the usual cues and programmatic routines that most
physicians were accustomed to, this kind of unit was unrecognizable

as an inpatient unit. This perceptual difficulty persisted until several members of the medical staff took their first trip to NYU's facility. The trips allowed a large cross-section of the medical staff to see the cooperative care concept in action. These trips really started the process of challenging our own traditional ideas about inpatient care.

The project then began to move from what had been called "Bruce's Folly" to one that required serious consideration. The oncology service was especially enthusiastic about Cooperative Care. One of the hospital's most frequent admitters stated that he would put all of his patients in this unit. That was especially encouraging, since prior to that action the particular physician involved never had publicly complimented any hospital administrative initiative.

Unfortunately, not all of the other services were as enthusiastic, and a few converts and curious observers do not translate into a successful new venture. The cardiology service did not see a place for their patients, and few surgical services were represented at the NYU facility. The project had many well-wishers but no medical staff champion. This is when the persistent administrative efforts began to pay off. A small group of physicians who had made the trip to NYU were so impressed by the patient and staff satisfaction with this mode of care that they stepped forward to actively promote this concept to the rest of the medical staff.

A Physicians Advisory Group was formed with representatives from several medical and surgical subspecialities. These included oncology, endocrinology, gastroenterology, cardiology, infectious disease, psychiatry, general surgery, ophthalmology, plastic surgery, urology, otorhinolaryngology, orthopedics, neurosurgery, and invasive radiology. The group began to meet regularly, and started to define which of the patients from each specialty might best be suited for admission to the Cooperative Care Center.

This is when the realities of real patient care and the Cooperative Care concept began to collide. Design features, from parking accommodations to bedside monitoring capability, became points of contention. Control of the patient record, patient autonomy, and the loss of physician and nursing control of the inpatient environment became threatening realities. Sustaining broadbased interest in the project often was difficult when these concerns were brought forward. In addition, individual departmental concerns often slowed the group's progress. However, with persistence from the committee leaders, the group ultimately was able to translate the needs of multiple specialties into an actual treatment floor design plan.

ROLE OF THE MEDICAL DIRECTOR

The next phase of staff development involved the selection of a Medical Director and a Clinical Director. Having achieved broad interest and a consensus on the generic cooperative care program, the next phase is highly dependent upon the skills of the medical personnel who will be responsible for actual program implementation. We began searching for these individuals with one committee charged with the selection of both candidates. Our thought was that these key individuals should be chosen from a pool of highly respected internal candidates who were capable of championing the project through its final stage. The selection process needed to be completed with enough lead time for them to develop a strong working relationship. They will then need to go to the target audience—physicians, initially—and begin developing the care protocols, department by department, physician by physician, for the most likely users. The Medical Director's role is crucial in building the confidence and enthusiasm that the medical staff will need to consistently use the Cooperative Care Center for a wide range of patients.

One of the goals of the Medical Director will be to expand the horizons of the unit, taking full advantage of its relationship to the teaching program of the Brown University School of Medicine. The unit should be an ideal site for outcomes research and other forms of health services research, in which medical students and resident physicians can be involved to the benefit of all concerned.

SELECTION OF SURGICAL PATIENTS FOR COOPERATIVE CARE

We envision using the Cooperative Care Center for three different groups of surgical patients. The first group will be those requiring hospitalization for treatment of surgical disease, while undergoing diagnostic evaluation. The second group will be patients who undergo invasive surgical procedures which necessitate short-duration postoperative care. These two groups of patients probably will receive all of their care within the Cooperative Care Center, as they require inpatient care but no direct continuous observation by nursing staff, as long as they are monitored and assessed by an appropriately instructed and supported care partner. The third group will be patients who have undergone major surgery and will be transferred to Cooperative Care from the main hospital for further postoperative management.

The first group outlined above consists predominantly of patients undergoing vascular and interventional radiology procedures such as arteriography, aortoiliac reconstruction with stents, and stenting for superior vena cava syndrome. Cardiac catheterization, myelography, treatment of renal calculi, renal or bladder cyst ablations, infusion of intravenous antibiotics, and ablative blocks for pain control are other examples of patients in this category.

The second group will be very diverse and cut across almost all of the surgical subspecialties (urology, otorhinolaryngology, orthopedics, plastic surgery, general surgery, ophthalmology, and neurosurgery). There is a subset of patients within each specialty who require inpatient care from one to five days following surgery and who, with proper support and care partner education, we predict will do very well in the cooperative care setting.

The third group above will consist primarily of neurosurgical, cardiac surgical, and orthopedic patients who will be transferred from the main hospital during their acute recovery from major surgery. For these patients, the Cooperative Care Center will serve as an intermediate step between the first days of surgical recovery and home care. We envision promoting this capability as an option regularly integrated into the care of these patients. We also anticipate that the cooperative care environment will be an ideal place for patient-controlled analgesia to be used.

In reviewing the number of patients from these three groups currently being treated at Rhode Island Hospital, it appears that there are at least 4,000 surgical patients each year who would be eligible for care there. If we assume that one half of those patients could find an adequate care partner, and that the average length of stay would be approximately 3–4 days, then at any one time at least 25% of Cooperative Care beds would be filled by surgical patients. This represents a different patient mix than that experienced at NYU, but underscores the potential and flexibility of this type of facility.

27

PRACTICAL IMPLICATIONS FOR INSTITUTIONS CONTEMPLATING THE DEVELOPMENT OF COOPERATIVE CARE

Bruce K. Komiske

Any institution contemplating the development of a Cooperative Care Center, or any other concept which is innovative and unique, must prepare itself for a long, difficult, and challenging process. Some of the key elements which must be in place for such an undertaking are:

1. *A strong CEO and board leadership* who are willing to encourage innovation and risk-taking;

2. *An institution which has clearly defined its vision, mission, and values*, and incorporated these into both a strategic plan and a facility master plan;

3. *A project champion* who is given the time and independence to research the field, identify best practices throughout the country, and define the project's scope and concept in a way which will captivate the imagination of the board, management, and professional staff;

4. *Competent consultants*, brought in as part of the team. These should include functional programmers, architects, financial consultants and, ideally, input from the hospitality field. When selecting consultants, it is critical that an appreciation for innovation and risk taking be considered.

5. *Site visits* to institutions throughout the country that have demonstrated vision and innovation; these also are critical to the success of a new venture. Ideally, the key members of the project team should travel as a group, photographing and documenting the elements of their tour both from the perspective of what they would like to incorporate and, equally important, those elements which do not appear to be successful;

6. *Strong leadership* from both the medical and nursing staffs, which is essential for success in any new patient care delivery endeavor. Without their leadership, support, enthusiasm and input, the development of a project such as a Cooperative Care Center is doomed to failure;

7. *Input from appropriate regulatory entities* such as the Health Department, other Certificate of Need approval agencies, and third-party payors. These key groups can be either strong proponents for an innovative, lower-cost alternative to traditional care or significant obstacles, who are interested in maintaining the status quo and resisting change at all costs;

8. *"Beware of the corporate immune factor!"* As a very traditional industry, the health care community will resist any significant change. To be successful, the project champion and all involved in the project must be tenacious and willing to follow their convictions during a long, slow process. It should be noted that the Rhode Island Hospital/ Women and Infants Hospital project went through two formal certificate of need processes and no less than 28 formal separate approval steps between the regulatory agencies and hospital board approvals;

9. *Models.* It is safe to say that without the model created by NYU and without their continued unselfish sharing and assistance, the Rhode Island Hospital/Women and Infants Hospital project would not

have become a reality. We hope to share the concept as developed on our campus, including any refinements in scope, architecture or program, as willingly with others as the NYU staff shared with us.

Equally important to key elements for success are some potential reasons for failure of the Cooperative Care concept. They include:

1. *Absence of a hospital license*: Although all of the third-party insurers and government entities generally support the concept of providing lower cost inpatient care in an innovative setting, without a license to operate, the reimbursement issue may remain uncertain until the facility actually is completed and contracts finally are negotiated. Very few boards can afford to take the risk that these arrangements will be completed prior to the start of such an ambitious undertaking. A good example of a project whose concept had merit, but which failed because of the lack of a license is the Temple Medical Inn in New Haven, Connecticut.

2. *Lack of critical mass of patients or beds*: It is important to understand that the Cooperative Care concept may not be appropriate or acceptable to all patients, and should only be considered as an option for a portion of the total patients. At Rhode Island Hospital/Women and Infants Hospital, for example, the 74–bed facility is less than 10% of the available beds. It would be difficult to conceive of a small institution allocating a majority of its beds to this concept.

3. *Contrast of facilities*: In our efforts to identify best practices, we became aware of several institutions that had attempted Cooperative Care on a limited basis in existing, renovated patient care units. As a result of low census, minor renovations and cosmetic changes were made to vacated units, allowing patients to share their rooms with family members. It is our opinion that a critical mass of beds, sufficient to support a separate therapeutic floor and the independence that would create, is a major factor ensuring success of this model of care.

MARKET RESEARCH

As noted in previous chapters, it is critical to talk to your customers prior to identifying a service for their use. Rhode Island Hospital and Women and Infants Hospital conducted extensive market research with its medical staff, existing inpatients, focus groups of former patients, and random phone calls to the community at large to firmly establish overall interest in Cooperative Care. Once the concept was clearly defined and the explanation of how it differed from traditional care was understood, there was overwhelming support for this unique alternative, and the hospitals developed a higher confidence level for its ultimate success.

MEASUREMENT OF SUCCESS

Rhode Island Hospital and Women & Infants Hospital have undertaken the development of a Cooperative Care Center with a clear expectation of documenting measurable success in seven key areas. They are:

1. *Enhanced patient satisfaction*: As part of our service quality effort, we have undertaken extensive surveys not only of our inpatient population, but of our employees, medical staff, and the community in general. We intend to track the survey response and compare comments received for traditional care versus Cooperative Care, with the hope that we will be able to demonstrate the value of the care partner and Cooperative Care concept.

2. *Lower readmisiion rates and improved patient outcomes*: Hospitals throughout the country are being held accountable to demonstrate improved patient outcomes. We are confident that, through tracking traditional patients, compared with cooperative care patients, we will demonstrate both a lower readmission rate and, ideally, improved patient outcomes.

3. *Fewer misadventures/incidents/errors*: Based on the NYU experience, we are confident that we, too, will experience fewer medication errors, and slips and falls than in traditional hospital units. This will, in large part, be due to the active involvement of the care partner.

4. *Increased job satisfaction and higher staff retention rate*: Based on preliminary feedback from the nursing staff involved in the planning process, it is apparent that the Cooperative Care setting is an ideal opportunity for nurses to do what they were trained to do, that is, provide medical support, services, and education, while eliminating the need to make beds and perform other nonclinical activities. This, we believe, will result in significantly enhanced satisfaction and retention rates.

5. *Lower length of stay*: Nationally, the average length of a hospital stay continues to decline. We anticipate that, with the preparation and education provided to the patient and care partner from the day they enter the facility, we will demonstrate a further reduction in

length of stay compared with similar patients seen in the traditional hospital setting.

6. *Lower staffing costs*: As a result of the use of care partners, we anticipate an operating cost of up to 30% less than that of traditional care. Our current staffing budget, based on the NYU model, demonstrates the ability to achieve this level of efficiency.

7. *Lower construction costs*: With assistance from our construction manager, Gilbane Building Company, we have been able to compare the construction costs for the Cooperative Care Center versus a traditional hospital. Our goal was to demonstrate approximately 30% less construction cost and, to date, we have been able to exceed that goal.

28

PROMOTING COOPERATIVE CARE

Florence S. Schumacher and May Kernan

Marketing of Cooperative Care at Rhode Island Hospital (RIH) and Women and Infants Hospital (WIH) began several years ago with the idea of a new service designed to meet the changing health care needs of the Rhode Island community. As the building nears completion, promotion of the new service is assigned to a preopening and promotion team. Marketing will be an ongoing function in the Cooperative Care Center, as the new service will need to continue to adapt to the needs of the two sponsoring hospitals and the Rhode Island environment.

UNIQUE CHALLENGES OF HEALTH CARE MARKETING

Much discussion has occurred among health care professionals about who makes the decision regarding hospital care. Market research has shown the growing importance of the patient, or "end user," in influencing what traditionally has been a physician's decision. However, the physician still remains the dominant decision maker. This is especially true in Rhode Island. In a 1993 Rhode Island Hospital study, sponsored by the hospital, 56% of physicians in its service area said they made the decision about which consulting physician to select; 19% said it was a joint decision by the physician and patient; while only 6% said the patient made the decision.

The appropriate promotional strategy for Cooperative Care is a "push" approach, where the physician serves as the key influencer in the decision of a patient to use the service. In contrast, if the Cooperative Care Center accepted self-referred patients, as the Emergency Department does, the appropriate strategy would be to "pull" the patient directly to the hospital. Today, third-party payors also have become instrumental in channeling where the patient is to be hospitalized, based on selective contracts with preferred providers. Traditional promotional strategies become irrelevant when a person's insurance does not allow the use of a facility. Hospitals must work directly with third-party payors to promote their services as well.

While all three groups—physicians, patients and payors—are important to promoting cooperative care, the initial key targets are the physicians, specifically the attending physician. Because the concept is so new to the region, many staff physicians are not yet aware of how they will be able to use the new facility. In order for patients to be able to accept their physician's recommendation, they also need to become comfortable with the new service. Once the concept becomes better known among physicians and patients, direct promotion to potential patients may become appropriate. The first promotional task, however, is to influence physicians to admit patients to the Cooperative Care Center.

A number of other audiences are relevant for promoting the new service. Initially, the focus will be on internal audiences of trustees, nursing and other clinical staff, nonclinical hospital staff and volunteers. Among external audiences, the initial focus will be on health care groups, such as third-party payors and particularly managed care organizations; local and state regulatory agencies; the academic community; and patient advocacy groups—especially the support groups for cardiac, cancer, and AIDS patients—who are expected to be major users. Other important external audiences include public opinion leaders, the media, and the general public.

POSITIONING

What benefits are to be communicated to the key audiences to convince them to use the new service? These benefits must be "positioned" next to the alternative to Cooperative Care, which is traditional hospitalization.

Despite the existence of the unit at NYU, cooperative care is not a familiar concept to the professional health care community and the general public in Rhode Island.

Fortunately, Cooperative Care is highly relevant to the major health care concerns of the 1990s. With increasing pressure from government and third-party payors to reduce health care costs, a major benefit to payors is that Cooperative Care has been shown to be as much as one-third less costly than traditional acute care hospitalization. A major benefit to patients is Cooperative Care's reliance on patient and family involvement in care and education about the illness, fostering patient empowerment. In addition, the modern homelike atmosphere will appeal to patients' interest in the amenities and hotel features of hospital care.

While these benefits also will be important to physicians, their initial concern will be that their patients receive quality care comparable to that provided on the traditional inpatient unit. NYU's experience supports that concern, but there is little hard data available to substantiate that Cooperative Care leads to reduced hospital readmission rates or fewer calls to physicians after discharge. Demonstrating such differences through clinical research will be a major selling point to physicians. Another important physician benefit of Cooperative Care is the strong collaborative approach among physicians and other health care professionals. Creating a convenient environment in which physicians can care for their patients will be critical to gaining their acceptance of the new facility.

The positioning of the Cooperative Care Unit, then, will be as a lower cost alternative to traditional hospital care, with the patients and families sharing responsibility for their care in collaboration with a team of health care professionals in a homelike environment that emphasizes patient convenience.

PROMOTING A NEW CONCEPT

The promotion of this new concept should move along the traditional marketing communication continuum of awareness, education, promotion, and trial. While most of the hospitals' staffs already are aware of the building of the Cooperative Care Center, there is little understanding among physicians and nurses about which types of patients will be appropriate for the new facility. Some staff members think of it as a step-down unit or a medical hotel. The first major task, then, is to educate staff physicians and nurses about the new concept in order to create preference for this alternative to traditional hospitalization and recommend admission to their patients.

It is essential that both physicians and patients be satisfied with their first experiences in Cooperative Care, because the best promotion will be their favorable reports. Monitoring satisfaction closely, therefore, will be another essential marketing component.

MARKET RESEARCH

While clinical research is a well established tradition in academic medical centers, market research is a relatively new tool. Measuring the effectiveness of promotional activity and patient and physician satisfaction through regular surveys will be important to a successful marketing effort.

To measure the success of promotional activities, it is essential to have a baseline for comparison. Since the initial key audience will be physicians, a survey of attending staff will be conducted prior to the Center's opening to measure their awareness and understanding of the Cooperative Care Center. This survey will be repeated at least annually .

Both RIH and WIH have surveyed physicians for a variety of planning initiatives, but regular monitoring of physician satisfaction with the Cooperative Care Center will be essential to identify and resolve problems early, especially in the first 3 months following opening. The method could be either a short mail survey or, preferably, a phone survey by a clinician from Cooperative Care, who should be empowered to resolve problems that are identified. Depending on the findings, the survey frequency might be reduced to quarterly for the rest of the year, followed by the annual physician survey.

It also will be important to measure patient satisfaction once Cooperative Care opens. While the hospitals have patient satisfaction surveys in place for the regular inpatient service, these questionnaires will not meet the needs of the new service. Initially, all patients in Cooperative Care should be surveyed to identify problems. After the first 3 to 6 months, the same survey used for traditional inpatients may be used regularly on a sample of Cooperative Care patients.

Patient focus groups also will be used to monitor patient satisfaction. These groups provide a qualitative way to assess the new service. The groups will meet quarterly to evaluate their experience. To assure adequate attendance, patients will be compensated for their time.

INTERNAL PROMOTION: THE FIRST TASK

By using a variety of approaches and working closely with the Medical and Nursing Directors, the promotional team will target the internal audiences first during the year prior to opening. Although there have been several educational events during the planning stage, the pre-opening activities will kick off with a major education program on the concept of Cooperative Care, for both the medical and nursing staffs.

On separate occasions, the Cooperative Care leadership team will present a slide show to the key internal audiences: Board of Trustees, Management Group, employees, auxillians, and volunteers. This targeted approach will continue with presentations to individual medical department meetings by the team to discuss the relevance of Cooperative Care to each specialty. These meetings should help to identify individual physicians who are interested in the concept, especially in those specialties that are expected to be major users; for example, oncology, cardiology, surgery, and infectious disease. They will be encouraged to become champions of the concept. One-on-one meetings with these individual physicians and the Medical Director will be helpful in this process. In these sessions, the physicians' concerns can be addressed in detail.

From these sessions, it is expected that a group of physicians will emerge who are "early adapters," i.e., those who are the first to catch the wave of a new trend and influence others to follow. These physician leaders will encourage other physicians to try Cooperative Care by their example. The promotional staff will solicit their help for public speaking or media appearances to provide "testimonial" communication as needed.

Department meetings will be held with ancillary departments as well, since their work will also be affected by the opening of the Cooperative Care Center.

An internal publicity campaign to build awareness and educate the nonphysician staff will begin about the same time as the above education programs. A "Cooperative Care Update" will appear regularly in existing hospital publications for physicians, nurses, and other employees. These will be written by the Medical, Nursing, and Executive Directors.

Prior to opening, a direct mailing that explains Cooperative Care and includes an invitation to tour the facility will be sent to all attending physicians and referring physicians. Direct mail will be used, as it appears to be the most efficient and effective communication vehicle to reach this audience.

This combination of formal and informal communication is expected to create the level of understanding required for physicians to select Cooperative Care for appropriate patients and recommend their admission.

PROMOTION TO THE POTENTIAL PATIENT IS CRITICAL

In order to be receptive to the physicians' recommendations, potential patients also need to become aware of and educated about Cooperative Care. The scheduled patient will receive information in three different locations: the physician's office, the preadmission testing area, and upon admission.

A brochure targeted to potential patients will be developed for distribution in physicians' offices for scheduled admissions and in the Emergency Department for unscheduled admissions. A videotape also will be created. The videotape will be shown in physicians' offices and also on the hospital's closed circuit television network, designed to serve transfer patients and as general information that all patients may view.

Patients who are scheduled for elective admissions will have an opportunity to tour the facility during their preadmission testing visit. At that time, a second brochure giving information about what to bring to the Cooperative Care Center and what to expect there will be distributed. Patients' expectations must be anticipated and addressed because their experience in the Cooperative Care Center will be different from what they would find during traditional inpatient hospitalization.

Once patients are admitted to Cooperative Care, they will find information in their room, similar to a hotel's service directory, about how to use the facility. Education for patients about Cooperative Care needs to begin before admission, so that their expectations will be appropriate and they will be satisfied.

PROMOTION TO EXTERNAL AUDIENCES

Perhaps the most important external audience is the media, since that is an essential vehicle to educate the general public. Prior to opening, the public relations staff will hold background informational visits for the media, and keep them up-to-date with media backgrounders and news releases as significant events occur. Especially now, when the public is so interested in health care reform, the cost savings and innovative elements of Cooperative Care will be emphasized.

Although the general public at large is a secondary audience, efforts to reach opinion leaders will begin prior to opening. Members of the Cooperative Care Coordinating Committee will give slide presentations to business organizations, such as the Chamber of Commerce and Rotary Clubs, and to patient advocacy and health care professional groups, during the 6 months prior to opening.

OPENING IS A KEY PROMOTIONAL OPPORTUNITY

The opening of a new health care facility offers a range of special event opportunities, with a formal dedication of the new facility the centerpiece of the preopening activities. While this will be an invitational event, it will be followed by private and public tours so that anyone who is interested will be able to visit the Cooperative Care Center before it opens.

Preopening tours of the new facility will be offered first to the major internal groups—trustees, physicians, clinical and nonclinical staff— and then to the external audiences via a community open house. These events will include self-guided tours, refreshments, mementos, and a pamphlet about the facility and concept of Cooperative Care. Through this first-hand exposure to the modern facility, with all its hotel amenities, the concept will likely sell itself.

In addition, the message will be reinforced through the media, who also will receive first-hand exposure to the facility with a special media briefing and a separate tour prior to opening. When the first patients are admitted, a media photo opportunity will be offered.

Opening events will be supported by paid informational advertising in the media. An "image" ad which promotes the innovative and collaborative aspects of the new venture has been used in business publications. In order to build interest among the general public, this ad will be modified and used in the months leading up to opening. Only through paid advertising can the timing and placement of the message be controlled. Although designed to reach a mass audience, advertising, like publicity, has a spillover effect on internal audiences as well.

ONGOING PROMOTION

Ongoing promotion will be needed until the identity of the Cooperative Care Center is well established and occupancy targets are met.

The marketing staff of the hospitals will continue to provide the needed promotional support to the clinical staff.

Particularly during the first year, the "Cooperative Care Center Updates" and other articles about the facility will run periodically in hospital publications. Various Grand Rounds and Nursing Rounds offer opportunities for the Cooperative Care Center staff to report on success stories, and internal communications will be extended to a wide external audience when appropriate special events or news opportunities arise. Paid advertising that highlights the patient and payor benefits of the Cooperative Care Center and the hospitals' leadership in this area will keep the new concept before opinion leaders and the general public. These formal communications will be supported by the informal communications of the increasing numbers of physicians and patients using the Cooperative Care Center. Their satisfied reports will be the most powerful promotion.

29

A PATIENT'S PERSPECTIVE

Doreen M. Hackley

One of my earliest memories involves being in a hospital. I was four years old and was having my tonsils and adenoids out. My family was gone and I was terrified. I still remember the ward and the smell and the nurse who wanted to take my temperature from the wrong end. . . . I was horrified at that and valiantly tried to explain that I was quite old enough to use a thermometer like a grown up. It was my first experience with surrendering my control—and my dignity—to hospital regulations. It was not my last. I have had many opportunities to experience hospital regulations in my lifetime, as a family member, a parent, a spouse and as a patient. It's ironic that I find myself working at a hospital . . . but maybe not. I've found a way to poke at the rules from the inside, an opportunity to make it perhaps a bit less formidable and frightening for someone else. For the past 2½ years I have been the "voice of the patient" as we developed our Cooperative Care unit at Rhode Island Hospital/Women and Infants Hospital.

The problem between health care providers and its recipients is that somewhere along the way they part company on the definition of "quality of care." Each would agree to technical competence as one of the key ingredients to this quality. To be truthful, however, I doubt many patients spend much time thinking about technical competence. It's taken for granted, sometimes unjustifiably. But technical competence is what I hear discussed when doctors, nurses and technicians discuss quality of care. Patients and their families talk about compassion—a doctor who comes in and sits down before he or she asks how you are, nurses who smile when they enter your room and take a minute to talk or answer a question, technicians who are thoughtful enough to make sure that you're covered and warm while you wait in a hallway for the transporter, residents who acknowledge you as a human being and not just an intriguing body part to further their education. I've experienced these providers of "quality of care"—though not often. In fact, in only one hospital of the seven I've "done time in" did they really understand the value of the human touch.

My memories of hospitals began, as I said, as a toddler. Over the years I've watched my grandmother and mother be hospitalized innumerable times, once concurrently, as they battled and succumbed to cancer. I spent more time than I care to remember rushing to emergency rooms with a sister who suffered a congenital kidney disease. I always felt like an intruder. Didn't anyone understand that I was entrusting them with my most valued possessions?

Imagine how I felt when I started having medical problems myself. Unlike many people, I knew what to expect, and it only increased my dread. And now here I am, 13 surgeries and twenty-something hospitalizations later, having survived cancer, but more important, having survived seven different hospitals, innumerable procedures, callous doctors, harried and rude nurses, less-than-human residents, indifferent and sometimes incompetent technicians, sloppy service providers, and deteriorating facilities—here I am working in a hospital.

I hasten to add that all the doctors were not callous, nor all the nurses rude, etc., etc. But enough of them were, and even one is too many. So we find ourselves once again looking at the definition of quality of care—and endeavoring to redefine it, combining the technical and the emotional, competence and caring.

The implementation of Cooperative Care will have an impact on more than just the facility in which it will be housed. I believe that as this concept catches on—and it will, if only for economic reasons—it will have an impact on the way we provide health care at every level. Consider the basic premise of Cooperative Care: patients and their care partners work with doctors and nurses towards their recovery, learning and taking responsibility for their treatment, reading and contributing to their records, administering their own medications, having someone close by to make sure they're warm and comfortable.

Be careful of the monster you unleash. Once patients and their families experience this quality of care they will never accept anything else. No longer will they accept being treated as diseased organs; no longer will they allow themselves to be talked over, ignored, examined in hallways and waiting rooms, left lying frightened and uninformed, asking questions and getting no answers, poked and prodded by gaggles of exhausted residents during predawn rounds. The manner in which we provide health care will change as the concept of Cooperative Care spreads. Although I would like to believe that my encounters with hospitals will be strictly occupational from now on, I'm glad for the change.

REFERENCES

Astolfi, A. A. & Wilmot, I. G. (1972). Cooperative Care Center will reduce cost of diagnosis, recuperation and education. *Modern Hospital, 118*, 96–97.

Balint, M. (1957). *The doctor, his patient, and the illness.* New York: International Universities Press.

Barker, J. (1992). Cultural diversity: Changing the context of medical practice. *Western Journal of Medicine, 157*, 248–254.

Bedell, S. E., Cleary, P. D., & DelBanco T. L. (1984). The kindly stress of hospitalization. *American Journal of Medicine, 77*, 592–596.

Belozersky, I. (1990). New beginnings, old problems. *Journal of Jewish Communal Service, 67*, 124–131.

Benner, P., & Wrubel, J. (1989). *The primacy of caring.* Menlo Park, CA: Addison-Wesley.

Berkman, L. F., & Syme, S. L. (1979). Social networks, host resistance, and mortality: A nine-year follow-up study of Alameda County residents. *American Journal of Epidemiology, 109*, 186–204.

Bernstein, L. H., Dete, M. K., Grieco, A. J. (1985). Are you ready for the new home care? Home care: avoiding institutionalization: Preparing for post-hospital home care. (Borders, C.R., ed.) *Patient Care, 19*, 20–67.

Brider, P. (1992). Patient focused care. *American Journal of Nursing, 92*, 27–33.

Brod, M., & Roberts-Heurtin, S. (1992). Cross-cultural medicine: older Russian emigres and medical care. *Western Journal of Medicine, 157*, 333–336.

Caroff, P., & Mailick, M. (1985). The patient has a family: Reaffirming social work's domain. *Social Work in Health Care, 10*, 17–35.

Chachkes, E., & Jennings, R. Latino communities: Coping with death. (in press). In B. Dane, and C. Levine (Eds.), *AIDS and the new orphans: coping with death*. Westport, CT: The Greenwood Press.

Chau, K. (1991). Social work with ethnic minorities: Practice issues and potentials. *Journal of Multicultural Social Work, 1*, 23–40.

Choi, T., Josten, L., & Christensen M. L. (1983). Health-specific family coping index for noninstitutional care. *American Journal of Public Health, 73*, 1275–1277.

Chwalow, A. J., Mamon, J., Crosby, E., Grieco, A. J., Salkever, D., Fahey, M., & Levine, D. M. (1990). Effectiveness of a hospital-based Cooperative Care model on patients' functional status and utilization. *Patient Education and Counseling, 15*, 17–28.

Cole, R. E., & Reiss, D. (1993). *How do families cope with chronic illness?* Hillsdale, NJ: Lawrence Erlbaum Associates.

Congress, E., & Lyons, B. (1992). Cultural differences in health beliefs: Implications for social work practice in health settings. *Social Work in Health Care, 17*, 81–96

Cooperative Care patient survey: Computer-generated statistical analysis of results. (1977). Unpublished data.

Cooperative care: Patients, partners, and professionals. (1981). *Geriatric Nursing, 2*, 338–344.

Covey, S. R. (1989). *The 7 Habits Of Highly Effective People*. New York: Simon & Schuster.

Council on Scientific Affairs, American Medical Association. (1993). Physicians and family caregivers: A model for partnership. *Journal of the American Medical Association, 269*, 1282–1284.

Creditor, M. C. (1993). Hazards of hospitalization of the elderly. *Annals of Internal Medicine, 118*, 219–223.

Crossman, L., London, C., & Barry, C. (1981). Older women caring for disabled spouses: A model for supportive services. *The Gerontologist. 21*, 464–470.

Culturelinc Corporation. (1991). Cultural factors among Hispanics: Perception and prevention of HIV infection. New York: AIDS Institute, New York State Department of Health.

Delgado, M., and Humm-Delgado, D. (1982). Natural support systems: Source of strength in Hispanic communities. *Social Work, 27*, 85–89.

Dillard, J. (1983). *Multicultural counseling*. Chicago: Nelson-Hall.

Dodge, D. S. (1993, February 20). Our breast cancer. *New York Times*, p. 20.

Donabedian, A. (1993). Continuity and change in the quest for quality. *Clinical Performance and Quality Care, 1*, 12.

Draft Document (1978). Program Development. The Cooperative Care Center of the Arnold and Marie Schwartz Health Care Center.

Echt, D. S., Liebson, P. R., Mitchell, L. B., et al. (1991). Mortality and morbidity in patients receiving encainide, flecainide, or placebo. The Cardiac Arrhythmia Suppression Trial. *New England Journal of Medicine, 324,* 781–788.

Eisenberg, L. A friend, not an apple, a day will help keep the doctor away. *American Journal of Medicine, 66,* 551–553.

Engel, G. L. (1977). The need for a new medical model: A challenge for biomedicine. *Science, 196,* 129–136.

Fowler, F. J., Massagli, M. P., Weissman, J., Seage, G. R., Cleary, P. D. & Epstein, A. (1992). Some methodological lessons for surveys of persons with AIDS. *Medical Care, 30,* 1059–1066.

Ghali, S. (1982). Understanding Puerto Rican traditions. *Social Work, 27,* 91–98.

Good, B., & Delvecchio-Good, M. (1981). The meaning of symptoms: A cultural hermeneutic Model for clinical practice. In L. Eisenberg & A. Kleinman (Eds.), *The relevance of social science for medicine* (pp. 152–164). Boston: D. Reidel.

Green, L. W. (1977). Evaluation and measurement: Some dilemmas for health education. *American Journal Of Public Health, 67,* 155–161.

Grieco, A. J. (1985). The kindly stress of hospitalization. *American Journal of Medicine. 78,* A78–A88.

Grieco, A. J. (1987). Preparing for home while in the hospital. In L. H. Bernstein, A. J. Grieco & M. K. Dete (Eds.), *Primary care in the home* (pp. 19–29). Philadelphia: Lippincott.

Grieco, A. J. (1988). Home care/hospital care/cooperative care: Options for the practice of medicine. *Bulletin of the New York Academy of Medicine, 64,* 318–326.

Grieco, A., Garnett, S., Glassman, K., Valoon, P., & McClure, M. (1990). New York University Medical Center's Cooperative Care Unit: Patient education and family participation during hospitalization: The first ten years. *Patient Education and Counseling, 15,* 3–15.

Grieco, A. J. & Kowalski, W. K. (1987). The "care partner." In L. H., Bernstein, A. J. Grieco, & M. K. Dete (Eds.), *Primary Care in the home* (pp. 71–82). Philadelphia: Lippincott.

Guendelman, S. (1990). Developing responsiveness to the health needs of Hispanic children and families. S. Clarke & K. Davidson (Eds.), *Social work in health care* (pp. 713–730). New York: Haworth Press.

Harwood, A. (1981). *Ethnicity and medical care.* Cambridge, MA: Harvard University Press.

Ho, M. K. (1991). Use of Ethnic-Sensitive Inventory (ESI) to enhance practitioner skill with minorities. *Journal of Multicultural Social Work, 1,* 57–68.

Holden, C. (1981). Health care in the Soviet Union. *Science, 213*, 1090–1092

Hulevat, P. (1981). Dynamics of Soviet Jewish family and its impact on clinical practice for the Jewish family Agency. *Journal of Jewish Communal Service, 58*, 53–60

Jacobs, C., & Bowles, D. (Eds.) (1988). *Ethnicity and race: Critical concepts in social work*. Washington, DC: National Association of Social Work.

Hispanic health: Time for data, time for action. (1991). *Journal of the American Medical Association, 265*, 253–255.

Kalish, R., and Reynolds, D. (1976). *Death and ethnicity: A psychocultural study*. Los Angeles: University of Southern California Press.

Kaufert, J. M., Green, S., Dunt, D. R., Corkhill, R., Creese, A. L., Locker, D. (1979). Assessing functional status among elderly patients: A comparison of questionnaire and service provider ratings. *Medical Care, 17*, 807–817.

Klarman, H. E. (1974). Applications of cost benefit analysis to health services. *International Journal of Health Services, 4*, 325–352.

Kristan, R. V. (1985). Cooperative care: Six years down a new path. *The NYU Physician, 41*, 52–61.

Kwan-Lorenzo, M., & Ader, D. (1984). Mental health services for Chinese in a community health center. *Social Casework, 65*, 600–609.

Lee, E. (1982). A social systems approach to assessment and treatment for Chinese American families. In M. McGoldrick, J. Pearce, & J. Giordano (Eds.), *Ethnicity and family therapy* (pp. 527–551). New York: The Guilford Press.

Lewis, G. (1981). Cultural influences on illness behavior: A medical anthropological approach. In L. Eisenberg & A. Kleinman (Eds.), *The relevance of social science for medicine* (pp. 151–162). Boston: D. Reidel.

Low, S. (1984). The cultural basis of health, illness and disease. *Social Work in Health Care, 9*, 13–24.

Mechanic, D. (1968). *Medical sociology*. New York: The Free Press.

Metzger, N., & Panter, D. (1972). *Labor-management relations in the health service industry*, Washington, DC: Science and Health Publications.

Minuchin, P., & Minuchin, S. (1987). The family as the context for patient care. In L. Bernstein, A. Grieco, & M. Dete (Eds.), *Primary care in the home* (pp. 83–94). Philadelphia: Lippincott.

Minuchin, S., Rosman, B. L. and Baker, L. (1978). *Psychosomatic families: Anorexia nervosa in context*. New York: Basic Books.

Mo, B. (1992). Modesty, sexuality, and breast health in Chinese-American women. *Western Journal of Medicine, 157*, 260–264.

Muller, J. & Desmond, B. (1992). Ethical dilemmas in a cross-cultural context: A Chinese example." *Western Journal of Medicine, 157*, 323–327.

New York University Medical Center evaluation of cooperative care center. (1985, September). Unpublished manuscript.

Oltarsh, V. (1991). Cultural bridges in health education. *Journal of Multi-Cultural Community Health, 1*, 12–16.

O'Malley, J., & Serpico-Thompson, D. (1992). Redesigning roles for patient-centered care. *Journal of Nursing Administration, 22,* 30–34.

Parsons, T. (1951). *The social system.* Glencoe, IL: Free Press.

Patient education plays integral role in innovative acute care unit. (1981) *Promoting Health, 2,* 4–6.

Planck, R. (1982). A center for cooperative care. *Interior Design, 53,* 212–213.

Poulshock, S. W., Deimling, G. T. (1984). Families caring for elders in residence: Issues in the measurement of burden. *Journal of Gerontology, 39,* 230–239.

Quality assurance study, cooperative care length of stay impact study, (1979, September 24). Unpublished manuscript.

Quinn, D. (1992). Principles of data collection applied to customer knowledge. *Journal of Healthcare Quality, 14,* 24–36.

Ransom, D. C. (1993). The family in family medicine: Reflections on the first 25 years. *Family Systems Medicine, 2,* 25–29.

Reiser, S. J. (1993). The era of the patient: Using the experience of illness in shaping the missions of health care. *Journal of the American Medical Association, 269,* 1012–1017.

Rivera, E. (1990). The role of the botanica spiritualist and santeria in the Latino community concerning HIV/AIDS. New York: New York City Department of Health.

Robinson, B. C. (1983). Validation of a caregiver strain index. *Journal of Gerontology, 38,* 344–348.

Rothman, M. L., Hedrick, S. C., Bulcroft, K. A., Hickam, D. H., & Rubenstein, L. Z. (1991). The validity of proxy-generated scores as measures of patient health status. *Medical Care, 29,* 115–124.

Rubenstein, L. Z., Schairer, C., Wieland, G. D., & Kane, R. (1984). Systematic biases in functional status assessment of elderly adults: Effects of different data sources. *Journal of Gerontology, 39,* 686–691.

Shon, S. & Ja, D. (1982). Asian families. In M. McGoldrick, J. Pearce, & J. Giordano (Eds.), *Ethnicity and family therapy* (pp. 208–228). New York: Guilford Press.

Sigel, I. E., Stinson, E., & Flaugher, J. (1993). Family process and school achievement: a comparison of children with and without communication handicaps. In R. E. Cole & D. Reiss (Eds.), *How do families cope with chronic illness?* Hillsdale, NJ: Lawrence Erlbaum Associates.

Sommers, A. (1971). *Health care in transition: Directions for the future.* Chicago: Hospital Research and Education Trust.

Sommers, A. (1978). Priorities in educating the public about health. *Bulletin of the New York Academy of Medicine, 54,* 37–40.

Sommers, A., & Sommers, H. (1977). A proposed framework for health and health care policies. *Inquiry, 14,* 115–170.

Stark, M. S. (1987) Heading home, prepared. *American Druggist, 196,* 53–54.

Sullivan, L. W. (1990). Healthy People 2000. The Surgeon General's Report. *New England Journal of Medicine, 323,* 1065–7.

Tagliacozzo, D., & Mauksch, H. (1972). The patient's view of the patient's role. In *Patients, physicians and illness* (p. 183). New York: The Free Press.

Valentine, K. (1989). Caring is more than kindness: Modeling its complexities. *Journal of Nursing Administration, 19,* 28–34.

Wadsworth, M. E., and Grieco, A. J. (1987). Diagnostic monitoring. In L. H. Bernstein, A. J. Grieco, & M. K. Dete (Eds.), *Primary care in the home* (pp. 139–153). Philadelphia: Lippincott.

Watson, P. M., Shortridge, D. C., Jones, D. T., Rees, R. T., & Stephens, J. T. (1991). Operational restructuring: A patient-focused approach. *Nursing Administration Quarterly, 6,* 45–52.

Wheat, M., Brownstein, H., & Kvitash, V. (1983). Aspects of medical care of Soviet Jewish emigres. *Western Journal of Medicine, 139,* 900–904.

INDEX